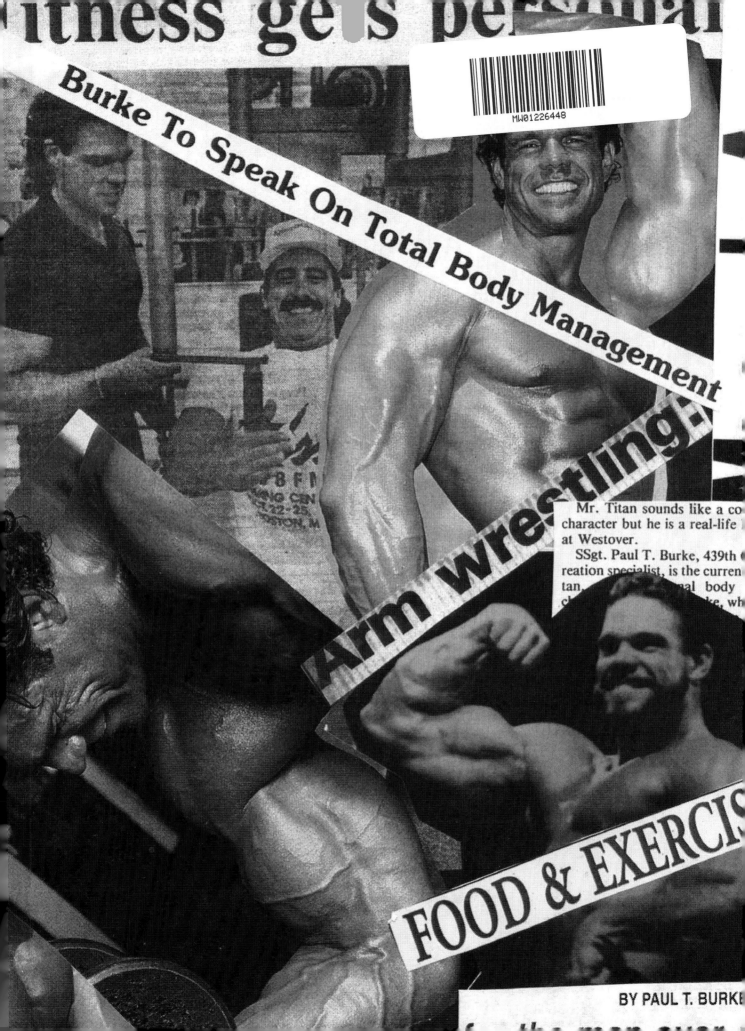

itness ge[s be[s[nal

Burke To Speak On Total Body Management

Arm wrestling

Mr. Titan sounds like a co
character but he is a real-life
at Westover.

SSgt. Paul T. Burke, 439th
reation specialist, is the curren
tan   nal body
c   ke, wh

FOOD & EXERCIS

BY PAUL T. BURKE

Note for Librarians: A cataloguing record for this book is available from Library and Archives
Canada at www.collectionscanada.ca/amicus/index-e.html
ISBN 1-4120-6939-4

Printed in Victoria, BC, Canada. Printed on paper with minimum 30% recycled fibre.
Trafford's print shop runs on "green energy" from solar, wind and other environmentally-friendly power sources.

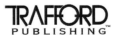

Offices in Canada, USA, Ireland and UK

Book sales for North America and international:
Trafford Publishing, 6E–2333 Government St.,
Victoria, BC V8T 4P4 CANADA
phone 250 383 6864 (toll-free 1 888 232 4444)
fax 250 383 6804; email to orders@trafford.com
Book sales in Europe:
Trafford Publishing (UK) Limited, 9 Park End Street, 2nd Floor
Oxford, UK OX1 1HH UNITED KINGDOM
phone +44 (0)1865 722 113 (local rate 0845 230 9601)
facsimile +44 (0)1865 722 868; info.uk@trafford.com
Order online at:
trafford.com/05-1850

20 19 18 17 16 15 14 13 12 11

BURKE'S LAW

A New Fitness Paradigm for The Mature Male

Paul T. Burke

Illustrated By
Theodore Cobb
www.vickicobb.com/theocobb.html

Table of Contents

Acknowledgements

Before I begin, I would like to thank a few people. Books are funny things; in that you end up writing the beginning after you have written the end. In reflecting on the writing process, it became clear who really deserves a public thank you. I have met so many people during this writing journey, and I would love to thank them all; among them, however, are four people who have propelled me to write this book, which is the culmination of my life's passion. First, I wish to thank my mother. She raised three tough boys by herself, and gave me the freedom of spirit and confidence to know that I could do anything I wanted to in life. And, believe me, I have!

Secondly, I wish to thank my girlfriend, Jodi. This beautiful, shrewd young lady has consciously and subtly led me to a place where I have become ambitious enough to tackle a book. Publishing a column for ten years was an easy groove to fall into; a book? Well, that is an entirely different story! Jodi, your love and support have made me want to be a better writer and a better man. This book is nothing more than our many conversations put into prose. Thank you, from the bottom of my heart, for making me want to be a better man.

Thirdly, is my one-time Boss and long-time friend Bill Koch. When I was in my mid-thirties I sailed with Bill Koch during his quest for The America's Cup. I also taught him how to work out and eat properly. He has paid me back in spades. Not only has Bill been a father-figure to me; but he continues to inspire me to reach above my physical problems and look for the opportunity within them. Had I never been diagnosed with MS; had I never ruptured my assessory nerve, I never would have sat down and put my knowledge on paper. Bill is an inspiration and he always seems to win. Thanks Bill…Thanks for the memories and thanks for showing me a way when I thought all doors were closed.

Lastly, I must thank my intellectual mentor, my philosophy teacher and my good friend Professor Chandler Steiner. Chandler passed away a few months ago due to a long painful illness. When I went back to school nearly ten years ago to get my Master's Degree, it was Chandler that lit up my nights traveling from Cape Cod to Cambridge, Massachusetts to attend a school that he helped make great; Cambridge College. We instantly became friends and he was another great mentor in my life. Had it not been for Chandler, the little, M. Ed. would not seem so real next to my name. Had it not been for Chandler, writing would be a frivolous exercise. He always asked me: "Is this the best you can do?"

To these two women and these two men, I owe a great deal of respect and gratitude for they all gave of themselves to help me get over hurdles that simply seemed too high to get over by myself.

Prologue

I learned early on that life is full of surprises, even more so, though, it is marvelously filled with magic. Each human body is magically diverse, and the key to success lies in mastering the tricks of each person's hidden talents – their own innate magic. As a member of a traveling circus and carnival as a teenager, I spent countless hours watching the magicians, sword-swallowers, geeks, "midgets," bearded ladies, strong-men and the other countless acts in the traveling shows. By doing this, I learned that everyone has a superstar somewhere within him or her. With no authority figure, school, or teacher to guide my experiences, I was allowed to figure out life and all of its mysteries for myself. It was in learning to find the "tricks" to any form that gave me the courage to name an ideology after myself. So, with tongue firmly planted in cheek, let us look at the history of strength, bodybuilding, fitness, and the principals that led me to devise Burke's Law. It is my pleasure to turn the fitness world on its nose; nothing would please me more than to reveal and change the tricks of the bodybuilding and fitness trade.

As you read this book, keep in mind – I do not have a superhuman genetic advantage over anyone. Like most people, I began training at a very average "starting point," therefore I have developed all kinds of unique routines to build up my body – rehab my body through countless injuries, which I will hopefully give you the correct knowledge to avoid ever getting injured; or, at worst, if you do get injured, know how to heal from the injury.

After building my body the "conventional way", however, I opted to abandon tradition and created a new, previously unheard-of training idea to win bodybuilding titles, naturally, without the use of drugs or harmful testosterone enhancers, Growth Hormone, insulin, or any of the other hundreds of pharmaceuticals that are now used to win titles in the sport of bodybuilding. Over the years, I have been able to put together the pieces of a massive physiological puzzle, discard the least necessary components, and put the rest exactly where they fit. Trust me on this -- I have learned the hard way.

When I was competing, I wanted to win more than anything I ever wanted to do, but as I got older, I realized it was actually the improvements that I was making that gave me the greatest satisfaction. You should try to remember when building a physique and staying fit, that it is all about you – not the guy who can bench press more; not the guy who can squat more; not the guy who has bigger arms: It's about you and how you progress and how you feel. No two bodies are alike, and therefore no one can try to catch another person in any area: The most you can do is maximize what your genetics have brought to you.

Winning is a great ideal; but it isn't the end. To quote the late great Vince Lombardi, *"Winning isn't everything; but trying to win, is."* As men in the middle or autumn of our lives', we must keep in mind that the goal is to keep ourselves in the best shape that we possibly can. Now, at age 49, simply being in good shape is a blessing, as I have MS and a great deal of severe nerve damage from approaching bodybuilding from a very foolish position. I was in the best natural shape of my life at age 44. Today, after four years of rehabilitating an injury that many doctors thought I would die from, I am once again in great shape. The human body and the power of one's mind and spirit are all unquantifiable. I honestly believe that anyone can achieve his physical peak anytime, even at age 60 or beyond. And muscles can certainly be maintained until the day you die. I want each of you to be saying these very words six to eight months from now, regardless of your age. Belief in oneself is as much a part of the process as the time spent on physical exercise and choosing the right dietary regimes.

Forward

By the age of 44, Paul Burke had made his mark as one of the most experienced and educated men in the fitness world. He had owned successful gyms, trained Bill Koch and had been the fitness equipment manager for Koch's winning America's Cup Team; trained celebrities all over the world, and had won many bodybuilding championships that spanned over three decades.

Equally amazing, during his mid-40's Burke possessed one of the best natural bodies in the world, especially when considering his age. He always spoke of "biological years" and "calendar years," and noted that they don't always coincide. Physically, Burke looked a decade younger than his calendar age and still does.

His ability to quantify and explain his own theory of muscle hypertrophy, fitness and nutritionally-enumerated calculations has established him as one of the most successful and long-standing columnists in our fitness and bodybuilding magazines. In this book, he now argues that building a muscular, lean, athletically functional body should take no more than 3-4 hours per week.

I know that Burke did not build his body with the help of supplements or other items that many seem to resort to. Burke wasn't "genetically gifted" either. He built his body himself, and has helped many others who sought and seek his help, all based on his eccentric view of the fitness world. His aren't difficult concepts to master, in fact, as Burke himself likes to say, they should "be obvious unless, one is blinded by his own layers of clouds falling down upon them like the past heroes of bodybuilding's glory days." In this book, Burke will teach us all how to utilize his theories, not only of how to build a great body, but also about the pitfalls of weight training. He is not afraid to admit his own mistakes, and speaks candidly about his own foibles, in an attempt to help others. I look to Paul's advice more than ever now that I'm past my own 40th birthday.

Steve Downs
Editorial Director, Exercise For Men Only, Men's Exercise, Natural Bodybuilding & Fitness.

Introduction
The Five Principles and The Way It Must Become

Before we get into the "muscle" of the book, it is important to understand the basic principles that I train by, those that I believe are the fundamental building blocks needed to understand my theories about lean muscle growth, fitness, health, functionality and longevity. These principles are set forth to make you think about how muscle hypertrophy and healthy muscular fitness are achieved. They will provide you with a vision for the perfect combination of mind, body, and spirit. It is important that you understand each of these Five Principles in order to reach your ultimate goals.

One:

You must perfect your form. Without a mastery of form, no results will be achieved. An awareness of your form during each exercise (and/or fitness activity) will cement the pillars upon which your entire fitness program will be built. The great artists of the Renaissance all had to learn how to draw a simple hand before they could move further into the realm of their own self-expression. Such a seemingly easy task takes great artists years; others may never accomplish the task. Which artist will you be? Will you be the artist who makes a half-hearted attempt at "form," or will you be the artist who learns and perfects the fundamentals, and then realizes your full potential?

In training with weights, maintaining proper form is biomechanically essential. As good form becomes second nature, you will be able to turn your focus toward mastering your perfect form. That which you find gives you the greatest leverage advantage in any given exercise; and thus be able to create Maximum Muscle Stimulation (MMS). That is, in weight training, the ability to contract a muscle and engage the greatest amount of muscle fiber in a non-stop, repetitive style, according to the demands of your body. Ultimately, it is your own perfect form that you must master. No one can tell you what your "perfect form" is; rather, you must consistently apply the training principals known to trainers and champions, and build upon them according to how they relate to the separate parts of your body. By doing this, you will be able to execute any fitness/martial art movement, and, in weight training, be able to focus on isolating each muscle, facilitating each part's individual growth. By doing this, everything will begin to flow together. You will be able to isolate muscles (or groups of muscles) to the degree that you will soon be able to contract and release each muscle until total fatigue occurs. To do this, you should contract and release the muscle as many times as possible without stopping, while supporting the greatest amount of weight that you can safely handle; contracting the muscles at an increasing rate, until fatigue occurs. In other words, you should be continuously shortening reps, feeling more intense contractions (you should not be stretching, or resisting slowly). Contrary to the standard idea that a "full range of motion" includes movements that feature a stretch all the way down, and then move the weight all the way up to contraction. You must find your own range according to each muscle group (your uniquely designed muscular-skeletal system), taking care to give the muscle its best chance for leverage advantage, which will then allow you to contract the muscle faster and faster to bring about muscle fatigue. Every muscle should be worked in this manner, in accordance with this principal, which I call, in part, "Burke's Law."

Two:

You must become aware of every nuance in your body. That is to say, you should devise your own routine, based on calculations in accordance with Burke's Law and its principals. You alone must determine when you should train with weights; how many sets should be done; how much rest to allow; how much cardio work to include in your regimen, etc. I will guide you through this process, and help you as you begin to build an entirely new, individualized fitness routine.

Three:

You must learn to stretch your muscles without forcing the stretch. You cannot stretch a muscle when lifting weights. People who tell you that you "stretch" when you go all the way down in a bench press, for example, are absolutely wrong. How can any muscle stretch under a load of weight? If you think about this logically, it would be like saying that you can jump the highest height possible with your arms wrapped under your legs (thighs). The best methods for stretching and relaxing weight-hypertrophied muscles are swimming, walking, Tai Chi, and yoga. Stretching on a mat after your work out may have some benefits, but it will not ensure sufficient muscle elongation or relaxation for someone.

Four:

You must eat in accordance with the calculations you will find in the nutrition section of this book. Eat nothing but lean free-range meat and Alaskan fish, lots of vegetables and a few fruits each day. Additionally, supplements of protein and creatine are often essential for muscle growth and performance. This book will explain to you how much protein, carbohydrates, and fats you should be taking in each meal.

Five:

You must sleep at least eight hours a night without interruption, so as to ensure proper REM sleep; fourth stage sleep. Proper amounts of sleep are needed to ensure muscle growth, fitness, elongation, functionality, health and longevity.

You must perfect these five principles in order to build and maintain a healthy, long-lasting, functionally durable and aesthetically beautiful body. But, before you can focus on your future, it is helpful to look at the past, in order to understand the origins of the health and fitness movement. It's incumbent for those of us who have gone the distance to turn around and shine a light for those on the path behind us.

Paul T. Burke, Master Educator

The Way It Has Become

Today, we take for granted the notion, that exercise is the path to feeling and looking good, gaining confidence, improving one's sex appeal, and for boosting energy levels. When exercise is approached from the right perspective, other benefits emerge, such as improved social confidence, an awareness of the goal-setting process, and self-confidence in achieving goals. In short, exercise has social value. Fitness has become an integral part of our culture; it has brought a new, heightened awareness of nutritional management and overall wellness into the culture at-large, and conventional wisdom has even accepted it as an effective way to remain psychologically fit.

Many people have approached fitness without the benefit of this knowledge, and therefore have reaped the benefits of exercise in a way they believed to be right, but which were not. Often, people who do stick with it, over-train, eat poorly (or neurotically), or take steroids. While these "cheating" and OCD (Obsessive Compulsive Disorder) type methods may give the temporary feeling and look of ultimate fitness, it is a flash-in-the-pan approach that can ruin and/or shorten one's life. In the short term, these methods are a terrible waste of time, energy and life force; in the long term, these types of ego-based endeavors prevent the user from learning the valuable life lessons of patience, vision and discipline. It is unfortunate that today's culture has decreed the outer facade to be more important than the inner soul. Many of those who exercise do it for the wrong reasons; but they will ultimately find out the hard way that their misdirected attempts at fitness, based on trying to attain maximum results by "cheating," will do them more harm than good.

As a lifelong athlete, bodybuilder, trainer, teacher and student, I have seen what happens when one chooses "easy" paths over "hard" ones; I have made my own mistakes, some of which nearly cost me my life; and yet, I have learned from them all. In this book, I will share with you the benefits of my experience. Here we will examine the origins of strength as a spectacle, follow it through the "fitness explosion" that transformed spectacle viewers into participants, and trace the rise of bodybuilding from the traveling carnival into the mainstream. Finally, I will outline what I call "Burke's Law." This is a new fitness paradigm, a new way of approaching what can be called "natural bodybuilding" and fitness for "Mature Men." As the saying goes, "knowledge is power." My knowledge has little power, however, unless I share it. Although books are sold, it is my sincere desire that each person who reads this book takes at least one idea from it and passes it along. This way, I will have given away more than I have sold.

1

History is The Best Teacher

Chapter One: Man Meets Iron

Man was designed for movement. Ancient man had to be strong, to hunt and kill his food, and to explore territories beyond his homeland. For cavemen and those living in pre-agrarian times, the notions of "exercise" simply did not exist; simple survival was the rule of the day. Life was strenuous and only the strong survived. Man rose up and out of nature, however he never has been, nor ever will he be, able to live without it.

Until the advent of plant and animal domestication, some 10,000-12,000 years ago, human beings, classified now as "neopaleolithic men," were hunter-gatherers. Males were traditionally charged with hunting for food, while females gathered wild berries, nuts, roots and other edible items. These tasks laid the foundation for our ancestors' health.

This was early man's way of life for millions of years. Their bodies evolved to include an uncanny combination of fast and slow twitch muscles that could accommodate both slow, heavy work, punctuated by quick bursts of energy (fast twitch) and, long, endurance-testing slow forms of motion (slow twitch). By today's standards, these early human bodies were, in their natural state, "super" athletic and "buffed;" they featured a biologically perfect ratio of fast to slow twitch muscle fibers. Neo-Paleolithic humans were tall and powerfully built, as compared to the hominid groups who followed over the next 10-12 millennia. Males and females who lived prior to the domestication of plants and animals had low levels of body fat and were able to utilize their unique muscle fiber combination to its maximum potential. Neopaleolithic man was the most muscularly well-balanced, athletic, lean, and symmetrical human group of all time. In short, they were "perfect" physical specimens. Today we know that the human body has the biological potential to live for 120 years, however we cannot hope to achieve this unless we live as close to the neopaleolithians as possible. Only by coupling their diet and exercise patterns with our modern comforts of shelter, sanitation, medicine, and even "stem-cell" research can we hope to reach our "natural" life expectancy.

As humans moved beyond the hunter-gatherer lifestyle, man's natural athletic ability to achieve high levels of strength and fitness began to decline. The notions of competition and combat remained an integral part of the human experience; however, they were increasingly acted upon out of pure entertainment. As a result, human bodies began to evolve away from the towering muscular form of the neopaleolithic era.

When tribal and territorial issues came to the fore, men had reason to "train" their bodies. The ancient Greeks and Romans built themselves up in order to fight in wars, to become gladiators, and to run long distances in the interest of communication. These efforts all pale in comparison to the physical conditioning of the pre-agrarian neopale-olithic humans, but it served these people well enough to continue a natural order in evolution.

Chapter Two: The Emergence of The Strong Man

In 1863, a large boy named Louis Cyr (pronounced "Seer") was born in St. Cyprien de Napierville, Quebec, a small town where the living was tough and the citizens both respected and competed with nature for their very survival.

Cyr grew up to become a lumberjack, a profession from which many "strongmen" have come. In fact, there are now "professional" lumberjacks who compete against one another for prize money. It is a far cry from the treacherous conditions and terrain of Quebec and other logging areas, but it has served to keep an old muscle-building, strength and athleticism tradition alive.

Legends say that, after days spent clearing the forest, Cyr used to visit the local black-smith, where the smith would perform feats of strength using his powerful forearms and shoulders. Cyr watched the smith carefully, and soon learned how to perform many of the smith's stunts and leverage techniques.

Cyr's reputation as a strongman was won early on. At the age of 14, he carried an injured lumberjack seven miles out of the deep woods during a snowstorm. Soon, however, Cyr left the lumberjack life behind him, moved to Montreal, and became a policeman. His experience in the forest served him well in his new profession, as he was able to handle those resisting arrest much the way he would have handled a trou-blesome log – one report even recalled how he carried two men under his arms to the police station, when they would not go with him peacefully. Logs, men, it made no difference to Cyr; he could carry anything, anywhere, no matter the weight. It was not long before a local newspaper dubbed him "the strongest man in the world." Word of Cyr's strength spread very quickly, and he became an overnight sensation. Cyr traded in his badge, and began traveling around Canada performing feats of strength and challenging all comers to duplicate his amazing abilities. In addition to other, stunts, he could be found lifting a platform holding 18 men on his back, and, in 1896, he set a record for lifting a dumbbell of 258 lbs. with his right hand while simultaneously hoist-ing 254 lbs. with his left over his head. Cyr picked up a weight of 552.5 lbs. from the ground using one finger, and could lift over two tons with his back. In one famed demonstration, he matched his strength against a team of four horses. With two horses reigned to the right and left of him, he was able to use his massive strength to stay his ground against the opposing pairs of horses. The horses were soon tired, and it became clear that they would not best Cyr. One horse collapsed, and Cyr was then called upon to help revive the worn out horse. Stories of Cyr's exploits pushing trains, lifting cement-filled beer kegs with one hand, and the like have been passed down, and continue to be told even in the present day.

The hubbub surrounding Louis Cyr's acts of strength created quite a fascination with the concept of "strength," and he was soon the toast of European society. Not only were the working classes intent on discovering his secrets, the wealthy were equally enthralled. Soon, rock tossers and log chuckers around the world were clamoring for a chance for similar notoriety, but Cyr's star remained on the ascendant. He traveled to Britain, then the world's greatest political and cultural power, and witnessed one of the oldest traditions of the British Isles, the Highland Games. The Scots had a long-standing contest of log tossing, wherein the competitor carried a log with two hands, heaved it straight up, and then released it to see how far it could fly. This was the sort of contest Cyr could really come to enjoy!

Too Much of a Good Thing

It is not only sad, but also predictable that the world's first strongman, Louis Cyr, was overweight. Standing 5' 9", he weighed 300 pounds, and ate constantly. Eating was more than a survival mechanism for Cyr; he force-fed himself to stay as large and "fueled" as possible, so much so that he ate beyond what his organs were genetically encoded to handle. He pushed his own physical limits ruthlessly, and soon his opponents became increasingly difficult to beat. As he aged, his growth hormone and testosterone levels began to decline. Louis Cyr, the strongest man alive, possibly the strongest who had ever lived, could not win the one, final, unwinnable battle waged by all men – aging. Louis Cyr died in 1912, at the age of 49. He had bested the strength of everyone in the world, and, in the process, eaten himself to death. In the end, his greatest strength proved to be the death of him. If Cyr's early demise can teach us nothing else, it is that anything in excess is deadly, and that this truism applied doubly in the context of weight lifting and shows of "superhuman" strength. Beware, my fellow fitness enthusiasts and weight-lifting friends, the more food you eat and the harder you push toward your goals, the faster you will burn out and die. This is an inescapable paradox.

A Discipline Defined

Around the time that Cyr was coming to prominence, an accomplished gymnast and weight lifter named Eugen Sandow began to draw attention to the aesthetic qualities of muscle, with the help of his well-balanced physique. Sandow regularly lifted barbells that held lead shot. [1]* By increasing the amount of lead, Sandow realized that he was able to build his already-muscular frame into an increasingly more defined one, and in

*Footnotes are on page 210

the process, became the world's first celebrity bodybuilder and strongman. Cyr was round and blocky, his muscles obscured by fat, on account of his obsession with over-eating as he attempted to beat all comers. He based his strategies on the simple principal that weight moves weight; yet, Sandow's body was that of a classic mesomorph marked by sinewy symmetry, low levels of body fat, and a classically-fashioned lifting technique developed through years of trial and error.

Measurement	Cyr at His Peak	Sandow at Age 35
Height	5' 9"	5' 9.25"
Weight	300 lbs.	202 lbs.
Neck	20"	18"
Chest	60" +	48"
Biceps	21"	19.5"
Forearm	16"	16.5
Waist	38 – 43"	30"
Hips	36"	42"
Wrist	9.5"	7.5"
Thigh	32"	26"
Knee	20"	14"
Calf	22"	18"
Ankle	10"	8.5"

Measurement comparison of Cyr and Sandow.

By comparing photographs and the joint and muscular measurements of Louis Cyr and Eugen Sandow, we find two very different bodies – ones that illustrate how dissimilar people using similarly disparate means can achieve very similar goals.

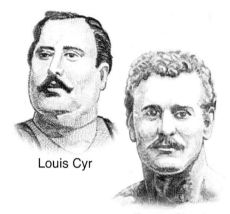

Louis Cyr

Eugen Sandow

What Cyr and Sandow Can Teach Us

Both Cyr and Sandow excelled by understanding and capitalizing on their individual body types and the capabilities of their individual body parts, in terms of leverage and anatomic design. When choosing a weight training routine, it is imperative that you, too, begin with this initial understanding. You must determine which of your body parts has the greatest advantage in terms of leverage, and then work to perfect your form when performing exercises with those muscles. Once you have determined your weaknesses, you will then be able to correct them by implementing the conditioning rules laid out in this book. Soon, you will be able to assess your strengths and weaknesses, and will know how best to address each of them, depending on bone size, muscle length, thickness and so on. In the chapters that follow, you will learn how to take the historic principles illustrated here, and apply them to your own life.

Chapter Three: Body Building and "The Average Joe"

Before we begin, I cannot emphasize enough that it does you no good to follow anyone else's weight training routine. In this book, you will learn to create your own routine based on the principles of muscular/skeletal measurements and leverage advantages/disadvantages that you possess. No aspect of weight training and muscle conditioning will be overlooked. You will come away from this book knowing everything from what exercises work best for wrists less than 7" in diameter, to how best to determine if your thighs have the potential to reach the impressive circumference of Sandow's thigh muscles, relative to his 14" knees. In short, you will learn that it is the circumference of one's adjoining joints that is the best predictor of a muscle's potential ultimate circumference. You will discover that one of the primary tenets of Burke's Law is that anyone, regardless of his or her genetic predictors, can build a great physique and enjoy lifelong functionality and fitness.

The keys to unlocking the power and strength that you possess lie in determining the most advantageous exercises for your body, and then perfecting and sticking with them until you can do them with ease. Breaking fatigue thresholds will become easier for you as you learn to stimulate the maximum amount of muscle fibers with the least amount of sets. This is a key element of Burke's Law: maximum muscle stimulation in the shortest amount of time. If you are content to be merely "average," listen to people who were once world champion bodybuilders, like Arnold Schwarzenegger and Lou Ferrigno. They and other successful bodybuilders were successful because they were blessed with the combination of great natural strength and nearly flawless physical frames. Most of us, however, have been graced with neither of these traits. So, what to do? We must approach strength training and muscle conditioning as analytic thinkers.

Burke's Law will help you to do this, and bring you the results that you desire. Make no mistake about it; you will need a tenacious spirit and an ability to maintain focus when faced with pain barriers. This is not a book for the weak of stomach, heart, or spirit; it is, however, a book that will show you, through historical examples, how to become the best you can be.

The traveling strongmen of old drew admiring crowds as they traveled the globe showcasing their amazing strength. Inevitably, onlookers began trying to duplicate these feats, but without any type of guidance, they had no way to learn what the strongmen knew: Could anyone match them? Or, was theirs a talent reliant upon some natural pre-disposition for strength? As time went on, these "wannabe" strongmen began to search each other out, and most often found their fellows wherever the carnival or circus had set up shop. Soon, these aspirants began to "train" for the next year's challenges. They developed "exercises" that they could practice on their own, and eventually began to compete with one another. Most of these early weight trainers held physically demanding, labor-intensive jobs; they were construction workers, steel workers, and blacksmiths. They were not strangers to discipline, or to physical challenges, and were accustomed to working long, hard hours. But, they had no sense of biomechanics; they had no concept of "training" as we do today.

Bodybuilding as we know it today grew out of the strength training methods developed by the early "tough guys" who sought to compete against traveling strongmen. However, it is important to note that bodybuilding itself is, and always has been, a different sort of endeavor than strength building. Bodybuilding, is a discipline that calls for a constant focus on pumping a specific muscle within a rigid form for each and every muscle group. Each exercise must feature a smooth, rhythmic quality, without the incorporation of any other muscles – muscular isolation is of the utmost importance; By contrast, weight lifting focuses on hoisting a given weight over one's head, within a form of sorts to be sure, but with more emphasis placed upon accomplishing the task at hand, than on the process, or form. **As we have discussed, in bodybuilding, form comes first. No matter which discipline you choose to pursue, you will benefit from moderate to heavy lifting, by gradually increasing weights; however, if you are concerned with building your body, the idea of lifting increasingly heavier weights to the point where you cannot maintain an idyllic, rigid form, you not only will be working toward a counterproductive goal, but also dangerous and foolish one.** As our bodies age, the joints will begin to suffer from "wear and tear." By lifting weights that are too heavy for your body, as defined by your joint sizes beneath muscles, tendons, cartilage, and ligaments, you will be doing yourself a dangerous disservice. These factors must all be taken into account if you hope to predict the potential shape and size of your muscles.

A Taste of What is to Come

The average man lives longer than Cyr and Sandow [2] did, therefore we need to be smarter and even more disciplined than they were; we must practice restraint and patience in our workouts, so that we can continue to train well into our later years. This is easy to read, but terribly hard to remember, especially at the gym when every man's testosterone levels are boiling over in foolish displays of the competitive spirit. If you stick to the rigid, you will win the race; you will slowly and methodically move to reach your own potential, and the raging rabbit will soon lie injured on the floor.

One thing that you should keep in mind at all times is that there are not three basic "body types," as the popular culture leads us to believe. On the contrary, there are hundreds of variations in bone, muscle lengths and strengths within every body. It is an oversimplification to say that some people are ectomorphs, and that others are mesomorphs, yet many training manuals will do just that, and then prescribe certain

19

exercises for certain body types, and others for other body types. Forget about describing yourself as a member of three all-encompassing pejorative metaphors.

Bodybuilding and The Masses

As World War II drew to a close, Americans were feeling more optimistic than ever before. California's sun and sand beckoned the war-weary masses, and a new hot spot was emerging, Venice Beach. Venice had a carnival atmosphere that attracted a certain number of free spirits, entrepreneurs, snake charmers and bodybuilders. One only needed to stroll down the beach to see bathing beauties, clowns, jugglers, artists, roller skating exhibitionists and lots of bronzed, men displaying their hard-earned muscles.

Among those drawn to Venice Beach was Joe Gold. He opened a small, mostly "free-weight" gym near the beach, in an area full of eccentric characters. Not far from Gold's Gym was another soon-to-be-significant spot, Vince's Gym. It would be at these two gyms that a man from Canada, who had been writing about muscle building, Joe Weider, began promoting bodybuilding in earnest. Soon, bodybuilders from all over were coming to Venice to train and tan. The "golden era" of bodybuilding was dawning.

The laid-back attitude of the day, the beautiful weather of Southern California, and its culture of circus-style spectacles combined to propel the pastime of a few into one that would soon attract the attention of the general public. The Venice Beach crowd was intent on displaying their bodies for all to see. Over time, three main schools of weight training emerged over this long period between the Cyr and Sandow era, up to the Venice Beach era. Joe Weider took inspiration from the past and began performing strength acts like those favored by his hero, Sandow, thereby taking these acts a step closer to what would soon become the new sport of bodybuilding. A second form of weight lifting, powerlifting, also emerged. Like strength acts, powerlifting could also trace its origins to Cyr's spectacular style. It features three types of lifts: the squat, the bench press, and the deadlift.

Finally, over-the-head lifting, as opposed to powerlifting, came into vogue, and was soon named an Olympic event [3]. Olympic lifting originally included three lifts: the clean & jerk, the snatch, and, until it was eliminated in 1972, the press. The International Olympic Committee (IOC) banned the press due to the rampant instances of cheating associated with the lift. Over the head lifting has one chief goal – to lift the weight over the head. This task is easily judged (although not so easy to complete), and therefore was conducive to the Olympic arena. The moves of powerlifting, the dead lift, bench press, and squat, were harder to judge because cheating is simpler in these events, and locker room drug use was becoming the norm.

Chapter Four: The Bodybuilding Boom

Once bodybuilding emerged as a breakout sport, "personalities" also began to enter the public's consciousness. Steve Reeves (1926-2000) was the first. Reeves was tall, dark, and handsome, and was blessed with a symmetrical build and flawless bone structure. He was the very embodiment of what bodybuilding should have been about. He trained hard, ate properly, and used his body and his charisma to win both the amateur American Athletic Union's Mr. America title (the oldest bodybuilding title in the U.S.) in 1947, and the professional Mr. Universe contest in 1950. He enjoyed a modicum of popularity both at home and abroad. In Europe, where he was most prominent, he was able to break into movies with a series of "Hercules" films. In spite of his massive success as a bodybuilder, only a few followed his path. Most bodybuilders who came later had neither the time nor patience for the rigors of a healthy, mindful practice like that followed by Reeves.

Arnold Schwarzenegger was the last, and only, bodybuilder after Reeves who was able to take his success and translate it into other arenas. The period after Reeves' success can be identified as the time when bodybuilding and fitness, two pursuits that should always work in tandem, began to diverge. Schwarzenegger popularized the previously underground movement in ways that Reeves could only have dreamt. His Austrian sensibilities, coupled with his newly-adopted American "can do" attitude, had the effect of taking bodybuilding away from its carnival-grounds roots and brought the notion into the public's consciousness. His personal popularity skyrocketed, and gyms and health clubs began popping up everywhere. Soon, it seemed, everyone was following in the footsteps of those who used steroids and those who condoned steroids to permeate the sport. Once the world discovered this fascinating new pastime, its cache and novelty wore off as quickly as it had come. The idea of "fitness" became synonymous with people who trained with weights, ate healthily, and looked lean and trim. Further, anyone with big muscles was automatically assumed to be using steroids, and was deemed a "muscle-head."

Boom Turns to Bust

The bodybuilding boom was just that – a near simultaneous explosion of different sports all stemming from the feats of a few early pioneers. In spite of the common heritage shared by Olympic lifting, bodybuilding and powerlifting, harmony was not the rule of the day among the athletes. Olympic lifters exist in a realm unto themselves. They were instrumental in the IOC's decision to include over the head lifting in the Games at a time when other lifters had not even contemplated lobbying for inclusion in the Olympics. Powerlifters, too, are organized, and today are lobbying for Olympic status. Strict body builders, then, became the "lone wolves," the ones that seemed to carry a chip on their shoulder, the ones trying to emulate Schwarzenegger.

Unfortunately for the sport, and the more these men tried to be like Schwarzenegger, the more his legend grew, and the further away Mt. Olympus seemed from everyone. No account of the history of bodybuilding would be complete without a note about US Olympic weight lifting coach Bob Hoffman. Hoffman was among the first people to sell pamphlets that encompassed two different disciplines, in his case, Olympic lifting and bodybuilding. He was also an early promoter of protein powders. Hoffman was blessed with both an interesting character and interesting ideas, but his dream for combining Olympic lifting and bodybuilding never caught on.

Chapter Five: Building a Dynasty

The Weider Brothers and The Birth of "Training"

Without question, the credit for transforming the world of bodybuilding into a mass-culture phenomenon lies with no other men than Joe and Ben Weider. From the start, they were able to identify the most lucrative up-and-coming names in the sport, chief among them, Arnold Schwarzenegger, and then market the appeal of the highly trained body to average people. They could even point to their own success as a way to convince others that it could work for them.

The Weider brothers were two skinny Jewish boys from a rough part of Montreal in the 1930s, who were sick of being taunted, chased, and pummeled by neighborhood tough guys. Though they only had grade-school educations. They were resourceful enough to read a Charles Atlas advertisement that spoke to them, and 90-pound weaklings everywhere. They began with a $7 investment and the Atlas method, and went to work building their strength. They couldn't afford dumbbells or barbells, of their own, so Joe took a railroad axle and wheels from a junkyard, and used them. Soon the bullies backed off, and Joe began winning weightlifting competitions; his younger brother Ben was not far behind him. After a while, admiring audience members began seeking advice from the Weiders, so they wrote and began publishing a newsletter, "Your Physique." It was mimeographed, and sold for 15 cents. Within months, the circulation reached 50,000. The concept of "training" for the masses was born.

Joe soon began promoting bodybuilding competitions and dictating the very terms and exercises that would become the foundation for bodybuilding from that point onward. Business took off almost immediately, and the Weiders were able, based solely on an implied product endorsement from a muscular man in a photo, to build a stable of the world's greatest bodies. Each of the Weiders' athletes were signed to strict contracts that forbade them to align themselves with any federation or association other than the ones they themselves had formed, the International Federation of Bodybuilders (IFBB), which presided over both amateur and professional bodybuilding concerns, and the amateur-only National Physique Committee (NPC) Without a doubt, the Weiders held the world of bodybuilding in their iron grip.

The Weiders never lacked for publicity. They cleverly employed psychology when dealing with bodybuilding's up & comers, photographing them all and declaring them "stars." Soon, it was considered a great honor to be photographed for and associated with the Weiders. Ben concentrated his efforts on their publishing empire, and Joe became known as the "Trainer of Champions". They sold products and equipment, and virtually "owned" all of the rising stars, thanks to their ironclad contracts. They were untouchable. Regardless of the Weiders' efforts, bodybuilding remained mired in the "circus attraction" milieu; bodybuilders and strongmen were considered muscle-heads and freaks by many, and most contests were held in high school gyms or carnival lots. The Weiders dreamt of making bodybuilding a "respectable" sport, the only thing they lacked was the person strong enough to do it.

Training's Early Evolution

Joe Weider coined phrases like super-sets, tri-sets, burns, stripping, overloads, kick-backs, down the rack, split and double-routines as he went along. Through trial and error, he happened upon certain exercises that, with proper repetition, made muscles "pump" and grow. He wasn't an exercise physiologist, the profession did not yet exist when he was fashioning his weight training routines after Sandow's and others', nevertheless, his new exercises quickly surpassed the results he had gotten from Charles Atlas' Isometrics. Once he developed his initial set of exercises, he experimented with them and made improvements based on his observations of the bigger and better body-builders who came to Venice. He then named each of the exercises, giving them special names and special meanings. He used language to create a mystique, so that one had to be a member of his "club" to understand. These names that Joe devised came to be "official" names for bodybuilding movements, and were universally accepted. Just as important as this naming success, the concepts that Joe developed have also been universally adopted. Weider published articles full of pictures and special codes, all touting the methods used by his stable of bodybuilders. Those he was working with by this time included Larry Scott (the first Mr. Olympia), Dave Draper (aka, "the Blond Bomber"), and a young Austrian by the name of Arnold Schwarzenegger, who had been nicknamed ("the Austrian Oak"). Weider signed each of these men to appear in his magazines, which included "Muscle & Fitness" by this time. The articles featured not only information about the men themselves, but also detailed their training routines. The routines, of course, featured terminology created by Wieder, thus cementing even further his influence over the foundation of this nascent sport. A key component of the Weiders' fitness regime was the unpublicized use of anabolic steroids. In their zeal to obtain the greatest possible results, the Weiders recruited men from the Venice Beach gyms, and used them to test new routines and diets. Part of this training program included introducing athletes to doctors who would prescribe steroids. Whether the Weiders officially knew of this widespread steroid use is uncertain, but it didn't take long for people to note the benefits of steroids; soon it seemed that everyone was using them. As a result, a new physical standard, one that was considered impossible to achieve in a drug-free environment, became the model of the day.

Another important contribution of the Weiders' was their creation of the "Mr. Olympia." Until this time, the highest one could go in competitive bodybuilding was the Mr. Universe contest, which was strictly amateur. The Weiders saw a need for higher competition levels, so they invited each of the past Mr. Universe winners to compete against each other for the new Mr. Olympia title. Before the creation of this new title, the most anyone could hope for was to be on the cover of one of Weider's magazines. In addition to the glory associated with winning the title, a cash prize would also be awarded – this was the first instance where bodybuilders were given a chance to be paid for their efforts. In 1965, the first Mr. Olympia title and cash prize, $1,000, went to Larry Scott.

Though the $1000 purse didn't compare to the regular bonuses paid to professional athletes in other sports, it did put professional bodybuilding on the map. Weider's dreams had come true. He would never have the greatest body himself, but he did "own" those who would compete for the title of "greatest bodybuilder in the world." Without Joe Weider, none of this would have come to pass.

In spite of the success of the Mr. Olympia contest, bodybuilding has lost all possibility of becoming a legitimate Olympic, or any other type sport because of its dark reputation for rampant drug use. The drugs used today threaten people's lives.

Bodybuilding is no longer a sport or circus sideshow, but rather, often groups of dreadfully abused people who have found a seemingly legitimate outlet for their anti-social behavior. Not all bodybuilders fit into this mold; but many have taken on that role. Their abuse of drugs only fuels their narcissism, and ultimately, destroys their lives. The gym can be a wonderful place to learn about oneself, the interworkings of the body, and to form lasting bonds with others. This is how it should be used. We must all stay away from illegal drugs and use the gym and its positive aspects to enhance our lives and longevity.

The First Bodybuilding Stars

Both Joe Weider and Vince Gironda were competitive bodybuilders. Gironda enjoyed widespread respect for his early work as a promoter and gym owner, and for years, he helped Larry Scott train. It was Vince and Scott's great "softball" biceps and thick forearms that made the "preacher curl" famous. Scott and Gironda coined the term "Scott-curl" or what earlier pumpers once called the "preacher bench," so named because its position made the performer look as if he was kneeling in prayer. Scott's arms were truly magnificent – he had massive forearms and big, bulging "softball" biceps. He trained in the days before massive steroid use had become widespread - three pills a day and hard work, his training regimen, was considered normal.

To help put Scott's achievements into a more modern context, we can compare him to Arnold Schwarzenegger, who came along a few years after Scott. It can be argued that Schwarzenegger had the greatest pectoral and arm muscles of all time; but Scott had the thickest biceps and forearms. Their arm dimensions especially, (Biceps; Scott: 20", Arnold: 21") remain impressive even by today's standards. Arnold trained like a champion, but Scott was a true over-achiever: He approached training with a neurotic focus that propelled him to the top of the field. Unfortunately, his high-profile days were over before he could transform the $1000 he won as the first Mr. Olympia into something more permanent. I often wonder what went on in the mind of my first childhood hero, Larry Scott. Scott was soon eclipsed by Schwarzenegger's massive shadow, but that doesn't matter; he was the first Mr. Olympia and will be remembered for that pioneering achievement. Timing is everything in life, and instead of coming in on the tail-end of a world wide sport; Scott came along a bit too soon for critical acclaim by those outside of bodybuilding.

In spite of our earlier discussion of Scott's program for building his arms, based on use of the curl that now bears his name, the sad fact is that this reliance on a sole exercise only works for people fortunate enough to be born with the right proportions and natural gifts that Scott possessed [4]. No two people are alike – no two arms have identical tendon lengths and strengths, or muscle cross-fiber tissues. What Scott and Schwarzenegger achieved does not work for most people. This is why Burke's Law, can help you. It takes into account all individual bone girths, muscle lengths, amount of cross-fiber tissue in any one area, tendon strength and metabolic characteristics. Burke's Law will teach you how to make the most of what you have been given genetically, <u>WITHOUT USING STEROIDS OR ANY OTHER ILLEGAL PRODUCTS.</u> If you want a world-class body, you have to be smart, work for it and eat specifically. Taking steroids will lead you to nothing but trouble.

In Burke's Law, the knowledge of one's own body and its capabilities are examined, body part by body part, with each specific bodybuilder's individual characteristics allowed for and taken into account. But, before we can get into Burke's Law, we must continue to explore the history of bodybuilding and fitness.

The Little-Known Showdown

After Scott won two Mr. Olympia titles (in 1965 and 1966), a Cuban by the name of

Sergio Oliva won the next two. The big showdown for the fifth Mr. Olympia title, between the Austrian Oak (Schwarzenegger) and Sergio "the Myth" Oliva, was set. Schwarzenegger had been beaten only once before, by Frank Zane in the Mr. Universe contest of 1968, and he vowed never to be beaten again. But this new nemesis, the genetically gifted Myth, almost made him eat those words. Formidable and swarthy, the Myth possessed a mind-boggling combination of frame and muscle mass. It is no understatement to say that Oliva was the most gifted bodybuilder who ever lived. He had a tiny waist, a monstrous chest, back and legs, and enormous arms to match his huge calves and downright freaky muscularity.

What kept Oliva from developing into the "next big thing," as his nickname seemed to indicate he would? There are two possible answers. One is Arnold Schwarzenegger. Schwarzenegger took Oliva's Olympia crown away. Some say that Oliva was "robbed," both in 1969 and again in 1971, when he tried to reclaim the title from Schwarzenegger. Others contend that Schwarzenegger was not only magnificent, but that he wanted the crown more – he "stole" it with sheer confidence, stage presence, and style, the likes of which had never been seen before in the sport.

There is another possible explanation for Oliva's decline, too. Some have contended that the Weiders were racist – that Oliva's Cuban heritage cost him the titles. We cannot say whether the Weiders were racist or not, but we can note that, over the years, it was mostly white men and women who adorned the covers of Weider's magazines. It is also interesting to note that the great Lee Haney, an African-American who broke Schwarzenegger's record for the most Mr. Olympia titles, rarely appeared on the cover of Weider's magazines. Perhaps it was just an issue of timing for Haney, but years earlier, Weider made it known that he was looking for an ambassador for the sport to make his dreams come true, and it was known (in certain circles) that the ambassador needed to be both white and charismatic. In Schwarzenegger, Weider found his man, and was able to put bodybuilding on the map.

Schwarzenegger used every trick in the book to beat out the massive Oliva. Oliva was then left to fade silently away, while Schwarzenegger made his own dreams come true. Schwarzenegger is the most successful bodybuilder in history, but without a doubt, Oliva walked away knowing that, under different circumstances, he may have won one more Mr. Olympia. He was, in short, a phenom, the likes of which will never be seen again; and yet, Schwarzenegger was all that and then some.

In Schwarzenegger, the Weiders saw something that they did not see in Oliva – a gracious and entertaining ambassador for the sport, one who could help turn the relatively new pursuit into an enormous money maker. Schwarzenegger won five consecutive Mr. Olympia titles, then retired, announcing that an acting career, and possibly politics, was in his future. Schwarzenegger cemented his legendary status in the film "Pumping Iron." His charisma and boyishness, coupled with awesome physical and psychological capabilities, captivated everyone who saw the movie. Schwarzenegger's big break came when he was cast in a new series of films that followed the adventures of a warrior dubbed "Conan the Barbarian."

Though some of today's competitors may be bigger than Schwarzenegger, Oliva, or Scott, to be sure, both the natural progression of genetics and improvements in training techniques can account for some of this, but the specter of drugs such as Growth Hormone, insulin, and other chemicals only today's champions know cannot be ignored as new, younger, more pharmaceutically savvy athletes emerge. For many, the end of the Schwarzenegger era marked the beginning of the decline of bodybuilding as a sport open to all, including those who sought a naturally built physique. In the following chapter, we will examine the "old way" of training, and then set the groundwork for a new fitness paradigm, Burke's Law.

Chapter Six: The "Old Way" Sticks

Thanks to the movie "Pumping Iron," a whole new generation of fitness enthusiasts began congregating at gyms and mimicking what they had seen in the movies or in magazines. This influx of new people helped solidify the "old paradigm" of training. Though fraught with bad habits, rampant misinterpretation, and poor man's imitations of moves and routines, these "old ways" remain. The logic is; "if it's good enough for Arnold (in Pumping Iron) it's good enough for me." To this day, both bodybuilders and "regular guys" training to get in shape look to the pioneer magazines, like Weider's, Kennedy's, and Balik's. By doing this, however, readers never avail themselves of the massive amount of newer information now available about fitness and nutrition; they never realize that most of the books and training routines devised by "champions," were written by people on steroids; with great genetics. Furthermore, by reading the champions' personal routines, they are led to believe that each one will work for them. This is a lie! No one routine will work for everyone; this is why Burke's Law was developed.

If you follow the techniques detailed in this book, you can be successful without steroids. Anyone of any age can develop a muscular, lean, healthy body using these techniques. Others may fail in their quest for a better body, because they base their program on the ways of the "old paradigm." It is disturbing that so many of these original "old paradigm" theories and training ideas have hung on and become a part of the physical fitness lexicon. Among these outdated, antiquated notions, is the belief in the use of steroids, testosterone enhancers, GH, HGH, Ephedra and Andro. Too many people have done themselves harm with these items, mainly because they simply didn't know any better. There always is a way; there always is a better way; there always is a way that turns conventional wisdom on its ear and produces better results than any-one ever thought possible. Burke's Law is the way. I cannot promise you a mountain of drug-induced muscles; but I can promise you the best you, you could ever naturally hope for.

How The Old Paradigm is Unknowingly Perpetuated

Soon after the fitness craze exploded, people realized that, with just a minimum of training, they could become certified personal trainers, and make a lucrative living. The certification process was an easy one, requiring far too little training or real knowledge. Because the industry was relatively new, there were few people to conduct the certification classes; therefore most teachers were really nothing but retired bodybuilders and self-proclaimed fitness "gurus," all of whom perpetuated the old ways of training. As a matter of course, many newly-minted personal trainers adopted the bad habits of their teachers, and unwittingly spread poor quality information at best; and harmful misinformation at worst.

A paradigm shift was in order. As we all know, paradigms have tricky ways of entrenching themselves within cultures – shifts only happen as a result of outside forces. Burke's Law is just that sort of outside force of thinking. This chapter will outline how Burke's Law came about and how it can help you in ways that you never thought possible, simply because you have been stuck in the old paradigm.

In today's non-drug tested contests, it is not uncommon to see huge, bloated stomachs, swollen organs, oil injected into various body parts, implants, blocky, out-of-proportion builds, and painted flesh – Bob Paris, Lee Haney, Lee Labrada excepted – no one looks real whatsoever. These bloated, out of proportion contestants did not engage in a paradigm shift; they merely built on the old, and added more drugs to the mix. The goal of Burke's Law is to teach you how and why things work the way they do, and how to approach your fitness routine from a new and different perspective, one that will yield better results than those achieved following "old paradigm" techniques. Even better, Burke's Law will allow you to achieve amazing results in much less time than an old paradigm program would require, and more importantly, you will do it without resorting to illegal drugs.

To truly appreciate the fraudulence of today's professional bodybuilding look, and the practices required for attaining the look, one needs only to compare the bloated drug-enhanced monsters of today's professional ranks to the founding father's physique. Cheating, or experimenting with today's super-drugs can never match the natural, 100% hard-won beauty of Eugen Sandow's look. If your intent is to build a symmetrical, beautiful, healthy body, and to live a long, healthy life, the old paradigm and its reliance on enhancement drugs is your worst enemy.

What becomes of bodies that have been pushed to their limits, once age begins to triumph over ridiculous persistence? Those who have taken it to the extreme have become unwitting guinea pigs, and know the answer. I have lived long enough, made enough mistakes, learned enough lessons, and beaten far too many odds, therefore I feel obliged to pass on what I know. If you're willing to give up all pretense of being an authority, something many men are unwilling to do, I can spare you a lot of pain and disappointment.

To this point, we have focused our story on how fitness came to be as it is today; meaning entrenched in the ways of the "old paradigm." Now it is time to turn to the new paradigm, Burke's Law, to learn how making an investment of time and hard work can ensure good health well into your older years. History is, by definition, in the past. Now it's time to smarten-up, locate the brain, and feel the burn. From this point on, you will learn of the newest contribution to the evolution in the study of physique building, fitness, longevity, how to avoid injury and give yourself the gift of an old age that isn't full of pain. I have climbed the steepest mountains, done things the old way, wallowed in the depths of weakness and clawed my way back into peak form. To survive, I had to get smart. To thrive as a bodybuilder, I had to reinvent the norm, I had to discard all that I knew; I had to find another way. To find this new way of doing, of being, I had to start with my body. I learned what it could and couldn't do. Added together, this knowledge has become Burke's Law.

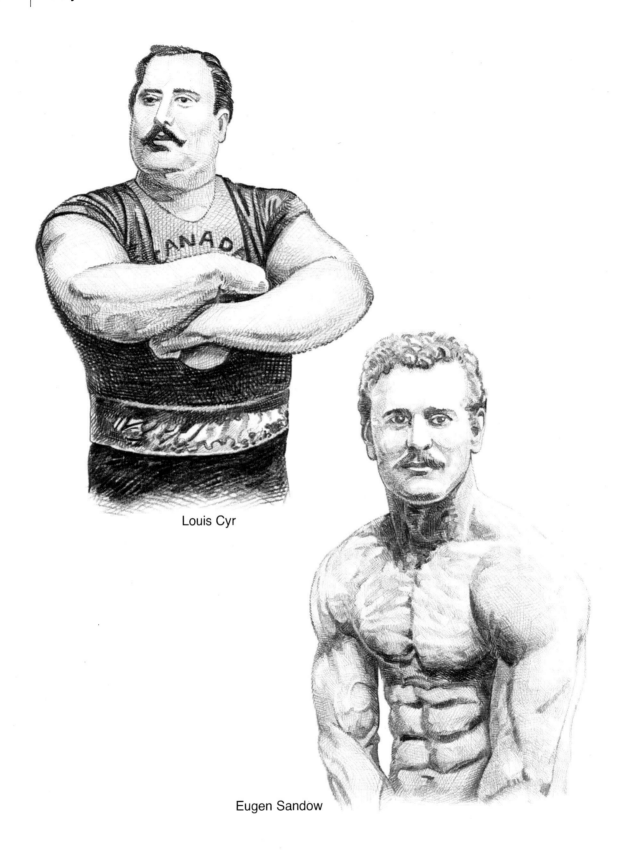

Louis Cyr

Eugen Sandow

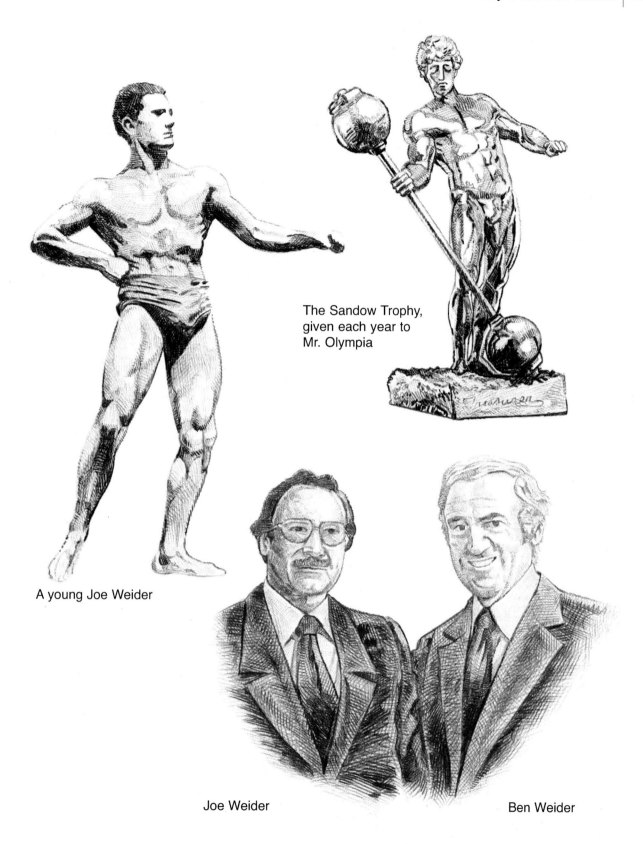

The Sandow Trophy, given each year to Mr. Olympia

A young Joe Weider

Joe Weider

Ben Weider

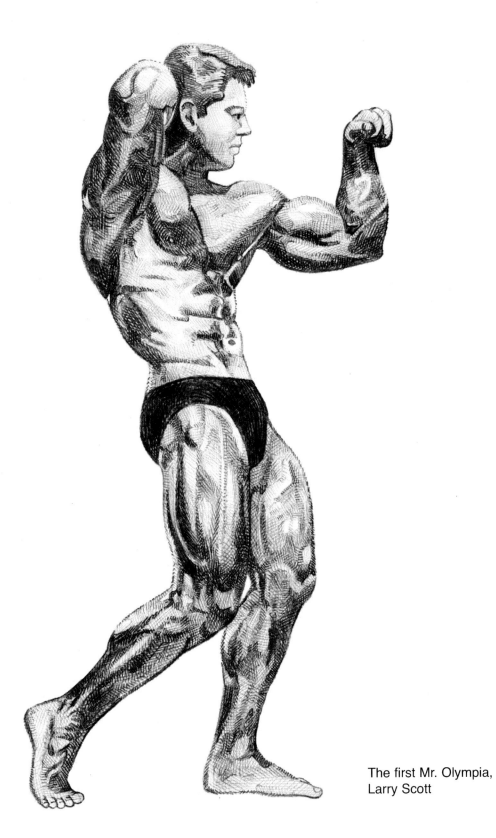

The first Mr. Olympia,
Larry Scott

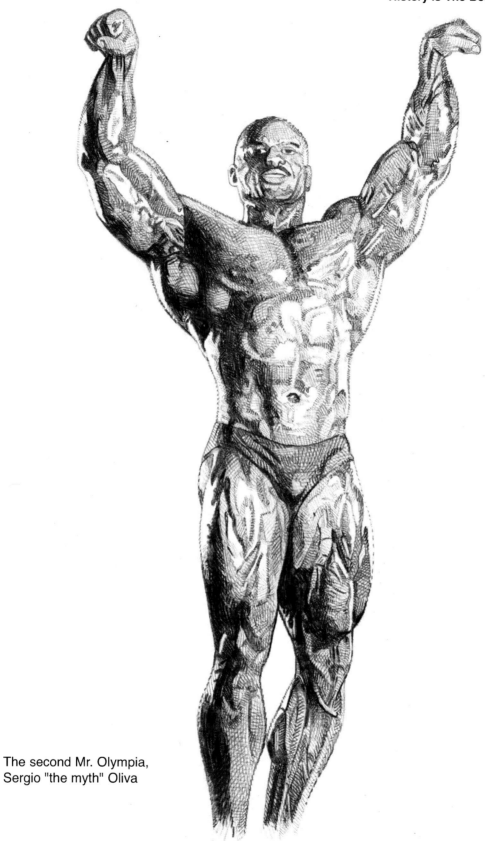

The second Mr. Olympia,
Sergio "the myth" Oliva

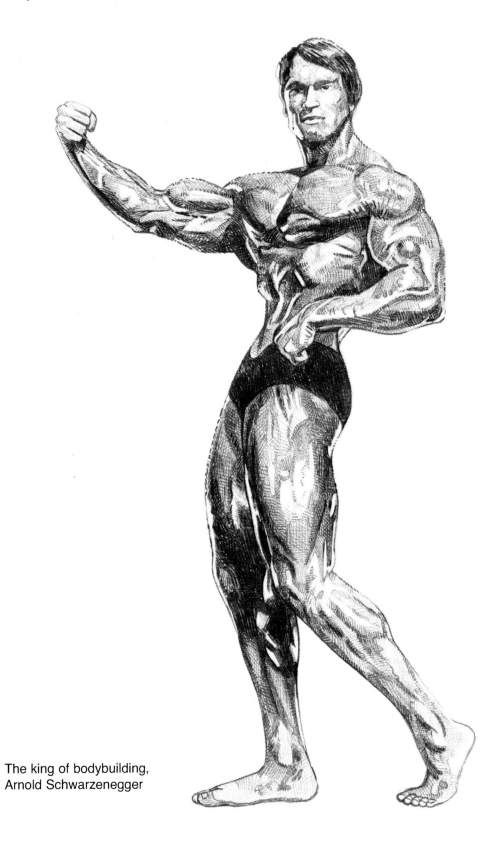

The king of bodybuilding,
Arnold Schwarzenegger

2 | Changing The Status Quo

- Structural Differences and a New Approach

- A Better Way is Revealed

- Forget What You Know and Start Where You Are

Chapter Seven:
Structural Differences and a New Approach

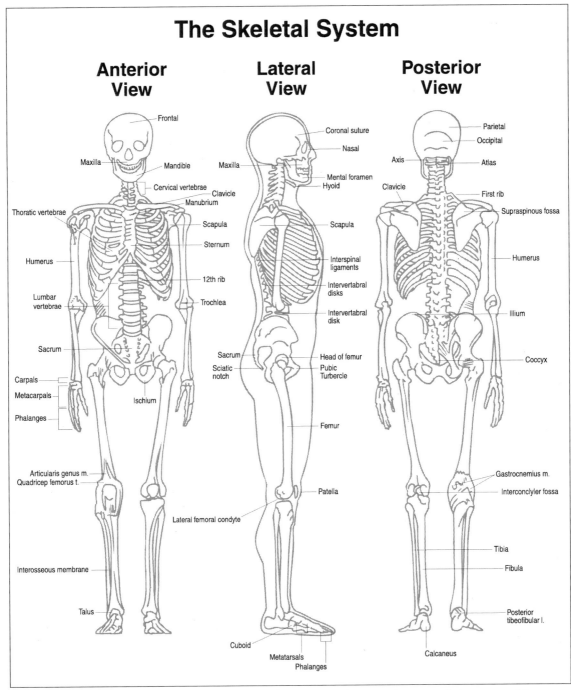

The Skeletal System

Despite the perfect proportions that every skeletal chart ever made presents, no one's bones are this perfect. Bone combinations are unique to everyone.

When I was in my late thirties, I knew I needed to shake things up, so I began to experiment. I tried working out fewer times per week; I went from working out up to six days a week, sometimes twice a day, to focusing on new exercises that I had made up, using them intensely but sparingly. I wanted to challenge myself to work towards a burning intensity, rather than focusing solely on stamina building and repetition that had the normal peaks and valleys that all bodybuilders thought was just part of the iron game. My criteria for success in this was to lift more moderately, focus on form, engage only in exercises that I did well, and eat in a way that allowed me to increase calories, yet still provoke muscle growth. My new way worked. It wasn't long before I had shifted my routine away from what I had read in Schwarzenegger's books, to what I knew would work for me, and maybe me alone. I had begun to realize that there was a natural answer for everyone, and that each answer would be different, given the different sets of questions each person would be asking.

By my early 40's, after competing in 31 bodybuilding contests (winning six, and placing in every one), I began experimenting with breaking the rules associated with the "full range of motion." I stopped counting training days, repetitions – even sets! I threw away my notebook and trained purely on instinct. These obvious departures from my usual fastidiousness surprised people who knew me to be a diligent record keeper and practitioner of traditional workout routines.

I had good reason to begin thinking outside the box. At age 41, I was diagnosed with Multiple Sclerosis. My world was turned upside down. While I was trying to pull myself together and get on with life, I found myself thinking of the early years when I spent late nights burning the candle at both ends, lifting weights in my parents' basement. In my late teens, I had developed perhaps the biggest forearms in the world, relative to my wrist size. This dramatic muscle development had come not only from genetic factors, but also from competing in arm-wrestling contests. I understood the arm-wrestling factor, but not the genetic aspect. Before long, I found myself questioning, "What is it about my forearms?"

After reviewing my records of past workout routines, days and weeks of experimentation followed. The answer to my first question was twofold: one, according to David P. Willoughby and George R. Weaver's pamphlet "The Complete Guide to Muscular Measurements," put out by The Weider Institute of Physical Culture, in Montreal, my wrists were quite large, relative to my ankles and knees. It also told me that my humerus bone was thick near the joint with the ulna bone. This information is significant because joint size is a reliable predictor of muscle growth potential. In spite of my intense forearm "workouts", it was actually my wrist and ulna bone that predicted the ultimate size of my forearm muscles; however, I had beaten the world record, and working the ulna's flexor and radial head had done it all. I accomplished this with both barbells and dumbbells, working until total muscle failure was achieved. Then, I repeated the process until my forearms felt as though they would burst had I done another set. In hindsight, it seems obvious to me that, if one's joints are relativity large when compared to other people of similar build, or to other joints within the body, these larger-jointed areas will grow easily, especially if the attached muscle is long and full. Burke's Law began with the realization that I could "grow" my forearms larger than the predicted size laid out by Willoughby and Weaver for those gifted with large wrists.

The second thing I took away from my unusual way to work forearms was a new understanding that to "grow a muscle," it must be contracted very hard, with only a millisecond passing before it is contracted again, and again, until failure. Allowing the muscle to relax will not achieve the results you are looking for. For example, someone with long arms and narrow shoulders should never do flat bench presses with a bar; by the time they execute the full movement, the muscle has been allowed to rest for too long. The biomechanics of this person's body isn't designed to compete with someone more suited for this type of movement. What to do? Use dumbbells, shorten the length of the repetitions; find a comfortable zone on a machine by shortening the length of pushing motion – merely an inch might do the trick. This, in essence, is Burke's Law: the notion that you should strive to move the most weight possible in the least amount of time possible, so that you can maintain a near-constant stream of muscle contractions. You will find this goal more challenging if you have not been blessed with large joints or a large cross-section or length of muscle fiber within a given muscle group, but don't be discouraged. As the old adage goes, "where there is a will, there is a way."

Nature Gave Us All a Slightly Different Physique

What Willoughby and Weaver had determined some 75 years ago turned out to be a vital key to my new way of thinking about bodybuilding. According to their theory, each joint is a basic predictor for attaching muscle size. Willoughby and Weaver focused their primary attention on the joints from head to toe and what the maximum attaching muscle could grow to each, without the use of steroids. They traveled worldwide collecting data from drug-free bodybuilders, and then were able to formulate theories based upon their findings. Willoughby and Weaver were among the first to provide important data for physique builders and their calculations became the standard formula for predicting muscle girth potential until the use of steroids. Few people even knew this booklet existed, but I never left home without it.

Formadal Structural Understandings in Burke's Law

Despite what Willoughby and Weaver did, which was lost years ago amongst the advent of steroids, there remains serious trepidations to consider before starting your own weight training and fitness routine. Here, I choose to discuss them, before I take you through to your own Burke's Law evaluation. The following are absolute necessities that you must look at.

Without question, the most misunderstood part about weight lifting is that very few people have ideal structures for training, while most simply don't. Oddly, even more misunderstood, is the fact that many people have actual structural deformities to some degree or another that can cause serious problems down the road while taking up a weight training program. Thus, they must be addressed before we move on. How do you know if your structure is slightly or seriously impacted by congenital malformation? And, if you are someone with a structural defect: what to do?

The most important part of self-analysis and/or the analysis of others is looking at the foundation of the skeletal system. Most important of all is the spine. Most of us believe our spine is "right" for our body; that nature couldn't have made a mistake – that our growing years were right for our body. Most of this theory is true; however nature didn't intend for everyone to be a weight lifter, a bodybuilder, a Martial Artist, etc. Walking around is one thing; lifting weights for years on end is not part of our evolutionary history; which brings us to the major malformations; how to identify them; how to correct them and how to work out with them.

Normal	**Kyphosis**
Diagram A	Diagram B

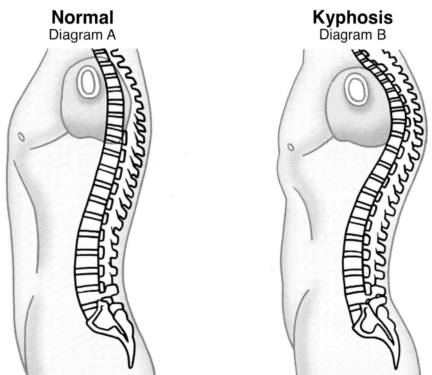

From this diagram we can see how a kyphotic back actually effects shoulder and chest development because the shoulders are already rolling down and forward and the back muscles are more stretched, not holding the shoulders and scapulas back. Any and all chest and shoulder development will make this problem worse, see deformities for full details.

In weight training the spine plays a huge role; and certain muscles can change the spine and other bones of the thorax because using good bodybuilding techniques; such as those I am outlining in this book, allows the muscles to begin to hypertrophy and they (or one in particular) pull in the direction where the most emphasis is; or, away from what might be called a congenital weight-training defect of the skeletal structure. For instance, the more someone is Khyphotic (see diagram on page 39), that being that the T-spine has an outward bulge and curves sharply back into the C-spine, the more this person must work on squeezing his scapulas together (and swim the "free-style" in order to straighten the spine and prevent a "winging scapula"). If this person doesn't do these particularly effective exercises for this congenital defect, this problem will not only get worse with weight training and/or age itself; it will end in possibly crippling injuries. Now, exercises such as low pulley rowing should be done with great form, and in a fashion where the exerciser is squeezing his scapulas together by bringing a bar that allows one to bring his elbows past the waist and really squeezing those scapulas together. A couple of easy exercises to do at home are to simply lock your fingers together behind your back, with your arms straight out, slowly move your arms upward; while another exercise is to simply hold your bent arms up at shoulder level and keep bringing them back further and further until you squeeze those scapulas together forty or fifty times at a time two or three times a day. Posture is key with this problem also. If you slouch and you have this problem, you will end up crippled if you train with weights moderately heavy for years.

If a person is weight training and has a Kyphotic back (known clinically as Kyphosis) and doesn't really isolate this rear muscular area surrounding the spine and scapulas, then he will end up with neck and shoulder problems when doing chest exercises. How? Why? Since the skeletal pre-disposition is already such that the spine is spreading the scapulas outward; and because of the roundness of the back, then any and all chest pressing (or chest exercises in general), if it is not countered with at least equal amounts of isolated work and intensity emphasized on this "scapula squeezing," then the tightness of the chest will pull the shoulders forward, causing problems with the sternocleidomastoids and the trapezius muscles. If indeed you inflame your sterno's (the two balanced muscles on either side of the neck), then quite possibly you can become partially, if not permanently imbalanced; or worse case—rupture a nerve coming out of your spine – feeding those very muscles. How? Let's talk about balance; pushing and pulling muscles that change the fundamental structure of the clavicles (or any structural part of the body).

First, let me say that over years, anyone can change his original structural form.

Let us go back to this rounded back called Kyphosis. If you have this, and you are building your chest and not isolating the back muscles to a greater degree, the development of the chest will tend to pull the shoulders forward, but at first, it will be so minor you will never realize it. Thus, not knowing how to approach this will lead to sure damage since almost everyone I have seen with this type of spine has rounded, slopping shoulders to begin with. This is probably due to a combination of the congenital structural problem and the tendency in childhood to find a comfortable position – which would be in a "slouching" position. Once this is your starting point, and since you can see your chest and tend to be able to isolate it better, then the chest and frontal deltoids pull the roundness of your back forward even more. You become more Khyphotic and more shoulder-rounded with each passing month of training. Eventually, over years, if the sterno's start to be disturbed by the clavicles (and the AC joints) change due to this growing problem, then your head will not sit perfectly still on your spine – especially when walking. Your sterno will fire at different times during simple locomotion and the brain doesn't get the normal balanced firing and then you begin to have vertigo, or a rocking feeling when you walk. I know this for a fact, because it happened to me. Since it happened to me, I have seen and helped two other body builders who were told they had Multiple Sclerosis (which I actually do have, along with a winging scapula and sterno imbalance). This, by the way, is crippling; you never walk straight again without having to look at your feet every step of the way. If you have any of these problems, be aware and follow directions closely.

To summarize about Kyphosis, if you even suspect you have it, and you are working out with weights, or plan to begin, remember your greatest weakness is in the very place you cannot see while exercising (the spine); however, you must try to pull your shoulders back by developing the trapezius and the smaller muscles such as the rhomboids; and you must use as many yoga and postural techniques you can learn; and swim as mentioned earlier. This, if it is a problem, you have to make a priority! You don't want to begin to work your chest until you have changed the spinal location from point (Diagram A) to point (Diagram B on page 39). Once your shoulders are in line with the less Kyphotic spine, then you can begin building your chest, never allowing it to become your focus only. Few, if any doctors or trainers on earth know these problems can even happen to a person lifting weights.

There are other exercises you can do to straighten your spine. Swimming, doing the free-style, or over-hand crawl, is a great way to straighten the spine because all of the back muscles have to work very hard to keep you afloat. Over time this will not only help your spine, it will elongate and loosen muscles – good for overall muscular-skeletal fitness, functionality and longevity.

Another way that seems to help this is to find a Feldenkrais practitioner and let them teach you some very subtle but strong neuro-motor reprogramming movements. This takes time, persistence, patience and an opening up to the awareness of your posture during the entire day.

Kyphosis, if seen in childhood can be corrected and it should be if at all possible. Many people with severe Kyphosis have trouble breathing, and live an older life in pain.

Lifting weights can be a big help here; but it can be as deleterious as a severe automobile accident if you follow a weight training routine blindly. Know your spine as well as you know your hand.

Scoliosis is another spinal abnormality and it can often be a deterrent to lifting weights. Depending on its severity at first notice, scoliosis may be treated with simple braces or operations not so dissimilar to those done on young people with Kyphosis. Basically an orthopedic surgeon places metal pins in certain areas of the spine and sometimes does some "reshaping" of bones. The outcome, if done early enough in life is one that usually will allow for any sports participation.

OK, now the question is: what if I'm forty and I've had scoliosis all my life – can I lift weights? This is a tough question to answer. I know I would recommend doing exercises on machines mostly, keeping downward pressure off the spine as much as possible. Again, swimming and Feldenkrais would be good therapies. Following a course similar to what I lay out later in the book, remembering not to put unnecessary downward pressure on the spine would be key.

When it comes to any type of deformity of the spine, whether it be severe, or slight, the best approach to getting at those tough muscles around the spine is to do exercises that squeeze the scapulas back and in; building a deep muscular crevice on either side of the spine and keeping your shoulders back at all times. The key is to remember that any exercise that does not squeeze the scapulas and tighten the lumbar are not for you if you have Kyphosis. Anything that puts large amounts of downward pressure is not good for scoliosis. There are various Pilates movements that are excellent for this type of frame also.

(Pilates: a systematic series of movements that helps the entire body, mind and spirit – Developed by Joseph Hubertus Pilates 1860-1967). This type of exercise was developed for the average person, but they are great for people with spinal malformations because many of the exercises require you to lie on the floor face down – raise the right arm and the left leg and hold; then do the opposite. Also, hyper-extensions help some with these problems because of their effect on crunching and thereby strengthening the lumbar area. As stated previously, swimming is supreme in this arena because it forces the back muscles to hold the body afloat. And, as mentioned, swimming also elongates other muscles because of the floatation of the body and the ease at which one can stretch, pull and thrust forward. If I had two exercises to do, and only those two, I would swim and walk – alternating days.

Chest Deformities That Must Be Reviewed

There are two extreme rib cage deformities that must be looked at before beginning any weight training program. They are; pectus carinatum, or "pigeon breast," and pectus exacavatum, or "shoe maker chest." These two deformities come in various degrees of exaggeration, much as the various degrees of kyphosis and scoliosis. The key is to know if you have a problem in this area because once again if you are weight training and you have one of these problems and do not address it properly, you could end up crippled.

There are many orthopedics that can build a brace for an adult with either such deformity, and over time, the deformity will lessen. Of course, surgery is a possibility here; but, I would hesitate to say that it is of all consuming importance assuming you have been living with this for 40 or more years. These types of surgeries should be left for people under 25 years of age.

These deformities should be looked at and examined before beginning a weight training program for the obvious reasons. The assessment of the deformity is key. If, for example, you have a minor deformity of the rib cage, then just keep in mind what I have already spoken to regarding Kyphosis and either of these congenital problems can be like a small snowball rolling down hill without the proper identity and the proper approach. If, however, the deformity is of great magnitude, there are braces to have fitted and very specific exercises to do. Find a very top sports medicine orthopedic in your area and be examined before beginning a weight training program if you suspect you may have a serious congenital problem in this thoracic area. Again, if you don't want to lift weights, or do other types of muscle building activities; then swimming and walking are the best. For most of you, awareness and understanding kinesiology are both important if you have any of these problems. You can follow my program; just adhere to the warnings.

There is one other comment I would like to make regarding the spine and the rib cage and their variations. Some people experience both chemical disorders and breathing disorders from any one of these malformations that I have mentioned. If you are experiencing breathing problems, exercise and braces will help, but surgery could be in order. Chemical problems are usually found in lack of Vitamin D, or not enough exposure to the sun; and/or, Vitamin K. All of this information, however, should be discussed with a specialist in this field before attempting a weight training program.

Hypermobile Joints and Weight Training

A hyper-mobile joint is one that can bend extremely in the "flexed" or "relaxed" positions; or act in hyper-mobility during normal use. Now, unlike the people with Kyphosis and Chest deformities, a person with hyper-mobile joints should focus on weight training and strengthening the joints by developing the muscles around it and not stretching or swimming as much. For example: there are people with high arches in their feet with the ability to pronate and supinate the foot in all four directions with ease. This maybe good if you want to be a ballet dancer; however, it would be imperative that this person not only work the soleus and gastrocneimius muscles of the calf with resistance training, but also walk long distances to strengthen the area in question in such a fashion that the ankle does not become easily broken, especially later in life. Hyper-mobility can be found in any joint, but wherever it is found, it should be addressed with symmetrical resistance training, coupled with some form of occupational therapy.

All of these problems exist in society, however they have never been addressed by the Weider's, or anyone else for that matter because they want you to think that if you take their products and follow their routines, then you too can become a "champion." What we all forget, but need to remember first, is that the people who have the greatest physiques are those who were given the skeletal structural stability, with the muscle mass – and thus could train like a "champion" to become one. I do not guarantee everyone a Mr. Olympia body; what I am doing, rather, is telling you all of the options available to all the different types of skeletal muscular male bodies out there.

You must learn to assess your own body and then follow along with this guide so that you can make the most of what your genetics dictate. Dream big, but be realistic in your assessment of how you are structurally, physiologically, and chemically. Therefore, before you begin to dive into Burke's Law, you have to identify spinal and structural problems and have them assessed (if severe) by an orthopedic sports medicine M.D.; or, a top-notch chiropractor.

Revelation

Back to our process of the changing paradigm in weight training. Once I set about analyzing my training style and experiences, all of the things I learned early on came flooding back, especially those young years while training for arm wrestling contests when I would do burning sets for forearms lasting minutes in duration. Once again, I began to think about my entire body as a group of interconnected fibers, ligaments, tendons, and bones. None of these fleshy, calcified parts of my body knew anything about "full" reps, or "sets"; nor would my body know the difference between my putting it through its paces with weights form a Nautilus machine or a rock in the backyard. Muscles respond and grow in very predictable ways – to intense, constant, sustained contraction while bearing the greatest amount of weight possible. There is nothing mystical about this process, let me assure you, but the founding fathers of muscle building – the very people we all looked up to when the sport was first getting started, were not thinking in this way. They were thinking about how Sandow and Cyr had lifted. Then they developed and believed in their own theories based on "full reps," "sets" "sets of 10 repetitions" "full range of motion," etc. These concepts were proven successful, as the full muscles of Larry Scott's arms, and the magnificent low hanging, highly muscled chest of Arnold Schwarzenegger can attest, but these practices only worked to a point (and usually worked best for those genetically gifted and/or on steroids). Without trying other ideas, however, everyone jumped on the Venice beach bandwagon, bought steroids, and used them. Some relied upon steroids for so long that they have been left with lifelong injuries and ailments. Others still have died very early deaths from them. Clearly, this was not a tenable solution. It was only through an open mind and willingness to explore other pathways that I was able to see beyond the old ways, and develop a quantifiable, successful plan for muscle growth and over-all fitness, Burke's Law. I was 45 and nursing a horrible injury, a ruptured assessory nerve. This experience taught me how to examine my life from a different perspective. Lying in bed for months allowed me to see muscles differently; how they grew well and how, and what didn't and why not. The "law" had been revealed to me. Now I share it with you. It will transform your ideas about training; I guarantee it.

Chapter Eight: A Better Way Is Revealed

As I have said before, I was systematically searching for a new, better way to train. I'd discovered the secret of contracting without rest to the point of muscle fatigue, and wanted to expand upon my theory, but was concerned. How, I wondered, could I do that with a leg press, or a bench press? It would be too hard to contract over and over, or push and push without stopping with the right amount of weight: Or would it? I began to experiment, first with full reps and heavy weights on the leg press. I began with a typical weight for me, at age 45, of 800 pounds and 12 reps. Though this is a respectable weight, I knew there was something within me that wanted more. My legs were shapely but not as good as my arms. By cutting the angle just a tad, raising the seat a notch higher to shorten the stroke, and adding a little more weight, I found a spot where I could get maximum fiber engagement for the greatest length of time at the highest velocity possible without losing stimulation in my thighs. After a few weeks I was sitting just one notch above my original position, but could, after only one warm-up set, complete one set of 30-35 reps with 1,200 pounds. I noticed that each week that my legs were growing, just as my forearms had when I was 12. I had found a place where everything "flowed" almost effortlessly. The burn and fatigue became a friend-ly feeling, and I only needed to do one or two sets; the main point was to be able to complete them without stopping. Once a set is stopped, progress, too, is stopped. There is so much more to building natural muscle than protein, carbohydrates, blood, pumping, and flexing. Once you are able to engage all of the muscle fibers for an entire set without stopping until you have achieved muscle fatigue, then you will have mastered the first principle of Burke's Law: Proper Stimulation; Maximum Muscle Stimulation (MMS).

My Formula for Forearms Revisited

My forearms measure over 16 inches in circumference, at rest. While I have benefited from a happy circumstance of larger-than-average arm joints, I still had to work to achieve this result. I did it by squeezing a bar and moving it only millimeters back and forth, contracting the muscles over and over, harder and harder, without even letting the bar go. I employed no "full range of motion," special rolling techniques, nor did I roll the bar down my fingers, the way that many trainers recommend. I did not count reps. I focused simply on moving the bar slightly back and forth, pulling it closer and closer, but always towards my forearms, for minutes and minutes at a time, until I could no longer hold the bar. This constant contraction is what mattered. This is all that is needed to stimulate the fibers properly. Your body components (oxygen, nitrogen, ATP, hormones, carbohydrates, water, calcium, potassium, sodium, etc.) will work together to help sprout muscle mass; but the stimulation must be done in the gym. The mental aspect of training is also important. Who among us hasn't seen contemporary photos of prisoners, for example, who may only eat two decent meals a day, yet look fantastic because they train intensely? They focus their few hours of physical freedom on intense, disciplined workouts. Much of their success comes from what no one can see – what goes on in their heads. This is a sport/art-form of inches and mind power. How can you, too, grow your arms to their fullest potential? You will do it by forgetting all that you have learned before, and by experimenting until curls feel "right," until you feel like you are doing something you were born to do and concentrate on it as if you were locked up, you had no other way to freely concentrate on your body. You must have a strong psyche, but a clever mind to go along with it. As I explained earlier, my forearms grew to world record size by following this simple plan of intense, burning, shortened rep, all out concentration on one specific muscle. What I was doing was totally off the wall. I moved the bar no more than an inch up and down. I produced increasingly hard and fast contractions, and didn't stop until muscle fatigue stopped me. I made a conscious effort to remember how this felt the first time I did it, and I now try to get to that same place with each body part. Once I conquer one muscle group, I keep at it until I cannot do another onset of the exercises. If you cannot get to a state of muscle fatigue, you are using too much weight, not enough weight, or perhaps the wrong exercise for the way that part of your body's joints and bones are configured. You must take care to get the biomechanics right – it is imperative that, as you are performing the exercise, your body be comfortable with the moves. If it is not, you will not be able to achieve proper stimulation because your focus will still be on form.

Can You Do It?

No matter what you have believed or been told in the past, everyone (structurally and physiologically able) can reach this perfect zone wherein they can move a heavy weight and engage their muscles until failure, without injury. The key is to find the proper leverage point, build up your anaerobic capacity, and keep going through the pain barrier, to achieve maximum muscle stimulation. Keep in mind, the bigger a muscle gets, the shorter it is, this is both good and bad. The shorter a muscle is, the fuller it looks, however with shortness also comes inflexibility. As years go by, our bodies can become truly distorted by this shortening of muscles. As muscles shorten, the myofascia begins to tighten, and bones begin to move in non-symmetrical positions (especially for those who have some spinal or thoracic deformity). This can have disastrous consequences. I myself ruptured my assessory nerve as a result of this process, and ended up losing my trapezius, teres, deltoid, and latismus muscles until my body slowly recovered over four years of pain, rehab, and a maze of doctors and PT's at my side every day. You will pay a price for distorting your body by lifting heavy and intense weights, but this is the very thing you must do to achieve maximum muscle stimulation. As you age, you must modify your fitness routine. Invest in and use rubber cables, learn how to stretch passively. You should stretch your muscles by swimming, Yoga, or walking, not by pulling or tugging on them lying on a mat in the gym. Pulling and tugging will only lead to an injury.

Keep in mind; muscle growth takes place after training. The most you can hope to do while at the gym is to stimulate more fibers than the last time you trained that particular muscle group. Afterward, you must eat in a way that will mesh with your workouts to bring about muscle growth. If it all works, which it will if you follow my plan, you won't believe the results. One other important concept to grasp: if you get to the gym and get into your routine and find that you cannot either match the weights and intensity, or surpass it, on any given muscle group: GO HOME AND REST. It does you no good to work out when you cannot make progress each training session. This is why you see people in the gym who look the same, week after week, year after year. This is a golden rule in Burke's Law: advance, or rest.

Now, at age 49, and because of the severe injury I had four years ago, I use Lifeline cables quite often mixed with free weights and cable machines. These rubber cables allow me to workout without hurting my nerve-damaged area. I use my own methods to get psyched up for the workout. My mind shuts everything out when I am training whether at home or in a gym. I look as good as I ever did because I diet precisely and focus on MMS. Therefore, I have developed a routine combining rubber cables and dumbbells at home, machines at a gym and continue to have great results. Using cables allows me to "pump" blood into tissues that have long memories. I can pull or push those last two inches repeatedly, so that a tight contraction and proper stimulation can take place. For anyone over age 45, I cannot recommend the use of cables highly enough as an adjunct, or a break from weights. They are powerful additional tools for your arsenal of training modalities, and they dramatically reduce the risk of injury.

As you age, you should weigh the advantages and disadvantages of weights and using rubber cables, or some of the less injurious home gyms that have come out recently that provide excellent range, resistance, and accessibility. Some people worry that they will not be able to build muscle with cables, or resistance type home gyms, but that isn't so. You can work every muscle and muscle group in your body with one set of cables and handles, or any of the very well constructed home gyms now on the market. It's all about form, focus and intensity (to reach MMS, and all about diet and rest to reach Maximum Muscle Hypertrophy (MMH). As we age, we must take care to protect our bodies from injury. By pounding heavy weights, the risk of injury is greatly increased, and recovery, as everyone knows, takes much longer once we are of a certain age. The methods outlined in this book do require intensity, extreme discipline, and constant concentration, but they will not cause you injury. In addition to cable training, I recommend swimming, brisk walking, Tai Chi, yoga, relaxation tapes, and similar methods to bridge the Western ideologies about building muscle with the Eastern ideas about breathing and stretching. All are valid, safe, and useful methods of exercise, breathing and stretching the muscles and keeping the spine loose. Just by lifting weights alone, your injuries can become chronic and even limb threatened. The lesson here is simple: if you feel pain, STOP IMMEDIATELY! Do not lift again until the pain has gone away, or until you have been to see a doctor or physical therapist. You may need light therapy to repair something; or you may need surgery to remove a bone spur or correct some other injury; whatever the reason, if you hurt, stop. It is my hope that you understand that, while Burke's Law is without a doubt the safest, fastest, most scientifically provable muscle building theory around, it, like all other exercise plans, does carry some risk. So long as you follow the "Rules of Motion" (outlined in Chapter 13), and you are able to understand this book in its entirety, you can reach your goals, stay fit, look and feel healthy longer. In the process, you will also be able to cut down the time you work out by a factor of .75. Most people will need to spend no more than 3 hours per week at the gym and two hours per week engaged in some other forms of "muscle lengthening" exercise, such as swimming, brisk walking, yoga, Tai Chi, or another martial art. One thing that I cannot stress enough is that you should not rely solely on "self-stretching" on a mat; or worse, with a partner pushing your leg to a point where something rips or ruptures. You should not stretch in the traditional, Western way of stretching only. If you are working out correctly, your muscles will be growing so quickly that you must use a form of exercise that stretches them as a secondary benefit; they should be stretched passively, not proactively or aggressively. Swimming is a good example of the type of stretching you should be seeking. In the water, your body weight is reduced; therefore your muscles can relax themselves and become elongated as you swim. Also, your back muscles must work hard to keep the spine afloat; and, perhaps more importantly, supple and flexible. If you force-stretch, or have someone else stretch you on a mat (especially if your body is cold), you run the risk of ripping a tendon or muscle. The worst thing you can do is bounce or force stretch when you are cold – not warmed up. Any stretching on a mat should be done after weight training; never before. Walking, if done properly, will also help your muscles to stretch. Tai Chi and yoga are wonderful because they allow you to get into anciently known positions that allow the body to relax and breathe properly, thereby allowing your muscles to lengthen and stretch and yet relax for life-enhancing breathing. Often times, even moderately heavy weight training makes one hold their breath; therefore, it is imperative to participate in a more "Eastern" approach to stretching (or swim as already noted). In my studies, the philosophical term for a person who learns the forms of the East and the West, to make routine right for their body would be called a "Triacic Self." This is truly a place to aspire to. The three dimensions have almost a plethora of subtle spiritual and physical meanings throughout history.

Each of these Eastern and Western disciplines takes time to perfect, but once you have achieved mastery, your muscles will relax and you will be able to continue to stimulate them to the fullest without the high risk of possible damage. This high intensity training is coined in Burke's Law as Maximum Muscle Stimulation with Maximum Muscle Elongation (MME).

Making The Most Out of Maximum Muscle Stimulation (MMS)

The late Mike Mentzer championed this type of highly contractive training for years, calling it "High Intensity Training," however he could not quantify and articulate a theory that people could easily understand. At the time of his death, in 2001, he was, I think, in the process of discovering many of the things outlined here. I certainly will remember him as having one of the most symmetrical and full physiques of his time. When Arnold Schwarzenegger made his comeback in Australia in 1980, few people who saw the show expected Schwarzenegger to place first over the very symmetrical, thick-muscled Mentzer. After he did, however, all hopes for bodybuilding's chance to be recognized as a "real" sport were dashed. Arnold made a rather half-hearted attempt at the Mr. Olympia title, this time as a promotional tool for his movie career. It backfired on him and, unfortunately, on Mentzer and the entire sport of bodybuilding.

Mentzer was the first man in history to score a perfect 300 in the Mr. Universe contest in 1979, just one year before his first appearance on the Olympia stage. His symmetrical, chiseled body astonished everyone as he walked on stage at the contest and took his place near Arnold Schwarzenegger, who at that time was only half the muscular marvel of his heyday. Schwarzenegger won, but the integrity of the judges was immediately called into question. Mentzer had been robbed, and responded by quitting bodybuilding forever. He spent his final years writing for Muscle & Fitness, but ended his life in a haze of drugs and alcohol.

Chapter Nine:
Forget What You Know, and Start Where You Are

There are times when we must all overcome our egos for the sake of practicality. It may not be the most appealing idea in the world, but if you want to remain in shape for your entire life, or just improve your odds for a functional lifestyle into old age, there are several things you must do.

First, you must forget about the century-old paradigms that suggest that bench presses with free weights are better than machines, that squats are the best exercise for legs, that heavy curls are best for biceps, etc. Use free weights, a selectorized weight machine, cables, or rubber cables – whichever one allows you to get the most leverage and force out your reps during the isolation process, so that you are able to achieve complete muscle failure for each and every individual muscle. The point is; no one way is right for everyone. You have to find your own way with the guidance of this book.

Next, you must learn about your body type and find the most advantageous exercises for each part of your body. By advantageous, this refers to leverage – the biomechanical structure that your parents have given you. You take it, analyze it, break it down, and begin to find where you are "locked in the groove." This then will lead to accurate individual muscle isolation and thus maximum muscle stimulation. I don't care if the biggest guy in your gym says you cannot develop a big chest without doing barbell bench presses: if the exercise doesn't suit you, another one will, and that one will build your chest better than if you fought yourself through injury after injury by doing the barbell bench press.

STEP 1:

You will be able to tell what equipment makes you feel the most powerful – free weights, machines, cables, or rubber cables. Wherever you feel the most powerful is where you belong, where your strength is – where MMS can be achieved, with smooth, rhythmic but difficult repetitions, one after another without stopping, without injury.

You should work each muscle group directly and with equal balance throughout the body. Focus on those two factors, and the results will astound you.

Your goal is to be able to continually work the muscle to the point of fatigue in one or two great sets. If you stop the flow of repetitions, you will actually reduce the intensity of the exercise, and therefore the potential for the greatest MMS. Counting reps is not a part of the MMS program, stopping for breath after eight or ten reps to reach twelve, then, is counterproductive. It is the intensity and consistency of the continual fluid reps and contractions to failure that matters. Take your muscle to a place it hasn't been before – **THAT BEING MMS**. MMS is the process that will burn fat and build muscle the fastest for the more muscle mass you add, the faster your metabolic rate, and you can burn fat while watching TV once you have everything working to perfection.

Stopping to catch your breath in the middle of a set can reduce the efficacy of your exercises by up to 50%. Keep going and reap the benefits of your hard work! REST ENOUGH TIME TO DO AN ALL-OUT SET. IT'S MOSTLY IN THE MIND DURING THE SET. MAKE EACH SET COUNT.

As Arnold once said; *"It's a case of mind over matter. If you don't use your mind, it doesn't matter."*

Once you have become skilled at MMS you only need to do anywhere from two to four total sets for your biceps or chest. You should choose a weight that is moderately comfortable when working to reach this intensity goal. Ultimately it is the smooth pumping motion and the intensity of the contraction that will effectively stimulate the most fibers. If the weight is too heavy you will over-tax your nervous system, ligaments, and tendons, slow down the constant contraction ability, and possibly injure yourself. Heavy, heavy weights are for powerlifters and Olympic lifters who struggle to complete one, or if they are in training, up to five repetitions. Truly heavy lifting is not appropriate for bodybuilding and fitness, especially when you are over 40.

It is amazing how small adjustments and minor changes in one's technique can make a tremendous difference in an exercise's outcome for the average person. People who are genetically gifted with favorable bone or muscle structure, or with certain metabolic advantages, will respond even better.

To maximize your natural potential, you must first know your own body. Second, listen to a knowledgeable, experienced teacher. And last but not least, do not accept hand-me-down routines or copy the top bodybuilders, who have genetic gifts or who are taking steroids.

Notes:

3 | Setting The Stage

- **Fit Over 40: Fact and Fiction**
- **Free Weights and Machines**
- **An Introduction to Burke's Law**

Chapter Ten: Fit Over Forty – Fact and Fiction

Common Misconceptions

1.) More is better, no pain no gain, one system fits all.

2.) There are only three body types.

3.) All the contraptions sold in TV infomercials have built the bodies of the actors selling them to you.

4.) It's a good idea to find someone with a great body and ask them to train you; obviously they know what they're doing.

5.) Special supplements and any old home fitness machine are enough to keep you in top form.

6.) After the age of 40, trying to stay fit is a losing battle.

7.) Anything is possible if you do enough reps.

One common misconception is that a strong, lean, fit, muscular body can only be achieved and maintained in one's youth. Many people would definitely consider such a physique unattainable for someone over 40. Conventional wisdom holds that only freaks of nature, with some magical genetic code infusing their body can achieve such a state in later years. In fact, nothing could be further from the truth. No matter what age you are and no matter what your genetic coding, body structure, muscle length, or shape, if you are reasonably healthy at 40 or older, with proper muscle stimulation, perfect form, training frequency, nutrition, adequate stretching of muscles and rest, you can build and maintain a strong, athletic, lean, beautiful body at any age. Muscle tissue responds very well long after the days of youth have passed. Many scientific studies have shown that men and women in their eighties respond to resistance training, and can increase their strength by as much as 150% in a matter of weeks.

These misconceptions about fitness can be traced to the early days of bodybuilding when people assumed that the best way to learn about building their own bodies was by copying what bodybuilders did, following the directions in bodybuilding magazines, and taking the supplements advertised next to the articles on becoming fit. In the early days of the fitness craze, these assumptions made some sense. It was an entirely new discipline, really not much more than a cult at the time; therefore very few scientific studies had been done on weight training or fitness levels.

According to the original guidelines for building the body with weights, as set forth by Joe Weider, Bob Hoffman, and Dan Lurie, one simply needed to purchase and follow their mostly-speculative routines in order to become fit. These routines typically required at least two hours at the gym every day and a high protein diet. The authors of these programs, of course, were happy to sell the requisite protein powders as well. Pictures of big musclemen holding the products were enough to convince customers that it would work.

The people who developed the industry nearly a half century ago, those who helped train or have themselves won the most important physique titles, have by and large, remained the "authorities" on bodybuilding. They continue to promote the old ways of building, and see no reason to change the system they helped to develop. The problem with this situation is that, oftentimes, these same people took steroids and most likely have compromised their current or future health and quality of life, all in order to be on top for a year while in their prime. Once past their prime, they have traded on their glory and begun selling things to you.

Those of us who have been around the physique and fitness world for decades, in the gyms, locker rooms, labs, libraries, and pump-up rooms, know the truth: you can build a great body and achieve tremendous fitness levels, with longevity in mind, in less than five hours a week.

Misconceptions about fitness over 40 don't end there. Some might tell you that no one over 40 has the cardio-vascular capacity, GH hormone or the testosterone levels needed to build your physique as well as someone in his twenties. This is partially based on the fact that testosterone and growth hormone levels diminish after the ages of 20 and 30, respectively. It is also understood that muscles, tendons, and even bones lack the strength they had during a man's late teens and early twenties.

You should not feel automatically stymied by these physiological "restrictions" without first having your hormone levels tested. "Normal" is a different number for everyone. Hormone levels are not necessarily a strong indicator for muscle growth potential. For example, I have had "low" testosterone my entire adult life, yet even in my mid-to late forties, my muscles respond very well. To understand how these hormones affect muscle development, you must examine the myriad hormonal, chemical, and genetic components that make up your body.

Planning to copy someone else's workout and expecting to duplicate their results is like asking a person who inherited a fortune how got they got so rich. Genetics has a big role in this.

Another misconception that has persisted from the "old days" is that you must spend hours in the gym each day and take thousands of dollars of supplements to look fabulous and feel good. The program outlined in this book will show you how to build a phenomenal physique, have great energy, reduce your risk of heart disease, stroke, and Type II diabetes, yet requires just five total hours per week in the gym, and/or at home walking, swimming, or engaged in one of the other appropriate passive muscle stretching activities. Additionally, good natural food from a reputable grocery store taken with a short list of vitamins and minerals is essential.

Many people assume that their calcium supplements are sufficient to prevent loss of bone density – osteoporosis and osteopenia, both of which are common consequences of aging. Training with weights gives the body a reason to retain more calcium and other vital minerals, therefore bones stay stronger and denser longer. If there is no biological need for increased calcium intake; the calcium supplements that so many people rely on end up being excreted, or worse yet, in areas of the body they never intended, like in the kidneys, in the form of stones. The longer you maintain muscle strength, length and flexibility, the longer you will be able to maintain joint integrity and skeletal density and flexibility.

Chapter Eleven: Free Weights and Machines

The fitness movement has been around long enough that most everyone now knows the difference between free-weights, and cables, rubber cables and machines, all of which in some way mimic the motions of the free weights, or dumbbells and barbells that the earliest bodybuilders used.

Cable pulleys bolted to walls at shoulder height and other such devices originated in the YMCA and Boys Club locations of the mid-twentieth century, and were designed to provide resistance to help improve the shoulder strength and punching power of boxers. Over time, however, others began to use the equipment, modifying then to work their arms, and later fashioning a way to perform "lat-pull-downs" and other such movements with the cables. You might remember the original "Universal Gym Set," which included at least one cable mechanism. This set was the prelude to many of today's weight-training machines. After the universal gym set gained popularity, new machines that mimicked other barbell or dumbbell exercises were developed to work the entire body. Nautilus was the first company to do this.

There are several attractive, practical reasons to use weight machines, and many companies, like Nautilus, Body Master, and Cybex, have capitalized on their user-friendly nature. Users appreciate machines, as they spare them the trouble of transporting dumbbells across the floor to a bench. With machines, the user merely adjusts the seat, places a pin to select the desired weight, and away they go. Today's equipment works every muscle of the body effectively and with relative ease.

What is important is to find which type of machine, bar, rubber cable, dumbbell, cable pulley system, or even bench that works best for each of your body parts, and then use it to its fullest. Focus diligently on your form, so that over time it will become ingrained in the memory of each of your muscles. Once your form has been perfected, you can turn your focus to intensity and increasing your anaerobic capacity.

A word to the wise: any form of resistance will do. Repeated, speedy contractions while bearing the most weight possible is all that matters in reaching MMS.

Chapter Twelve: An Introduction to Burke's Law

I have spent years working to move past all the consumer and politically-driven rhetoric of bodybuilding to formulate a unified, simple, scientifically-based theory for improved training results. That theory is Burke's Law.

Along with proper nutrition and ample amounts of sleep, exercise promotes the secretion of growth hormone (GH), a necessary ingredient for maintaining cellular integrity as we age. GH excretion also influences insulin production, which is also an important component of the aging process. Glucose uptake during exercise is a non-insulin-driven event, which is good news for anyone who has a genetic propensity toward glucose regulatory problems like hypoglycemia and/or Type II diabetes. Blood sugar used during exercise is consumed without insulin secretion.

Begin With The "Four Basics":

Make Your First Step a Giant One.
Learn How to do These Things Properly.

1.) Know your body and build each of YOUR muscles in accordance with your individual physical structure. No one's body is identical to anyone else's.

2.) Keep your body elongated and adaptable to all kinds of movement.

3.) Eat consciously, with knowledge about how foods affect you (covered in entirety in Section 9).

4.) Be a smart athlete: allow yourself to rest and recuperate.

Once you have mastered these basics, you will never need return to counting sets and reps or days on and off. You will have begun a training routine that's custom made for you. This, in a bigger sense, is where your strength is because you are a virtuoso at being yourself.

Notes:

Notes:

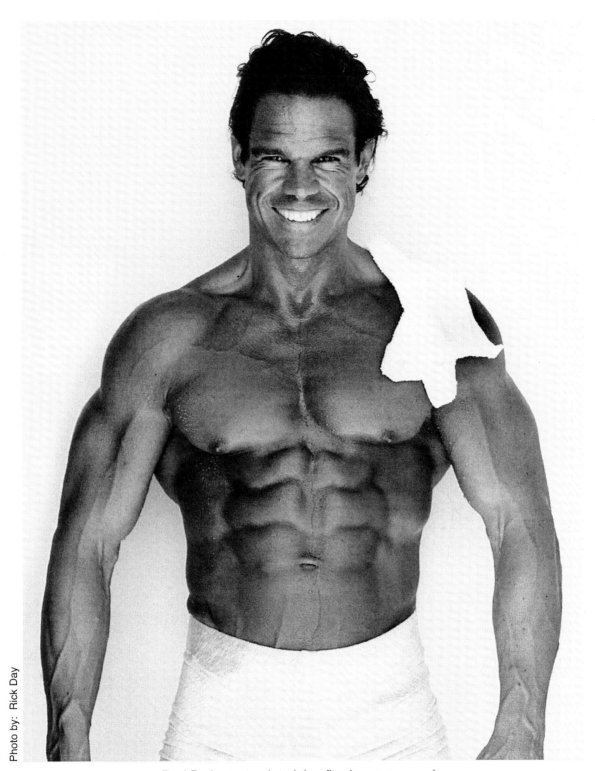

Photo by: Rick Day

Paul Burke, natural, training five hours per week.

4 | Burke's Law & Beyond

- Laying Down The Law
- Knowledge Is Power
- Identifying Strengths & Weaknesses

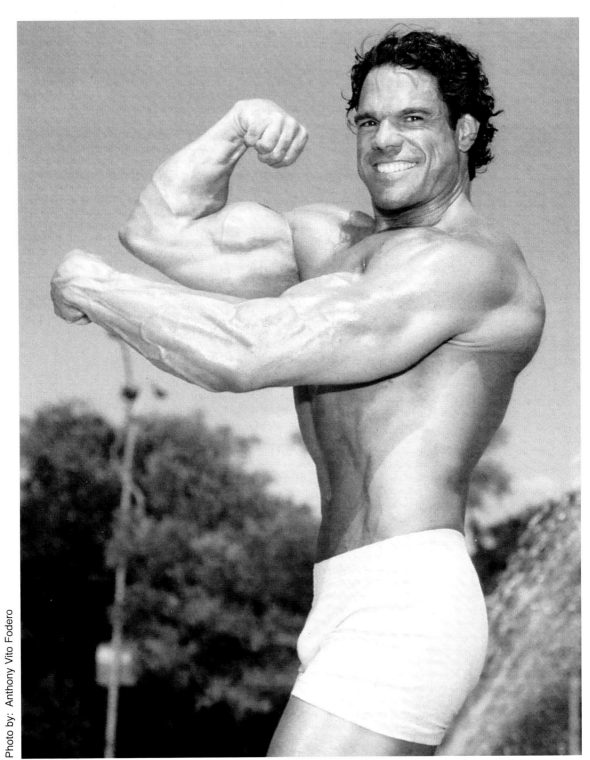

Photo by: Anthony Vito Fodero

The author at age 44. Natural, training five hours per week.
Photo: Courtesy of Chelo Publishing

Chapter Thirteen: Laying Down The Law

Building a fitness routine designed just for you and your body is not going to be easy, because you, like everyone else, are a creature of habit. Doubtless, you have been doing certain exercises certain ways, and planning your routine according to the amount of sets you do, how many days of the week you will train, what time you train, which exact routine you will do according to a schedule, etc. THROW IT ALL AWAY AND SET OUT ON THE ROAD TO MAKING YOUR DREAMS COME TRUE. One of the great aspects of the human mind and body is that it can learn something new at any time. You can reprogram your nervous and muscular systems with nothing more than determination, discipline and dedication.

Defining Burke's Law Scientifically

**MAXIMUM MUSCLE STIMULATION (MMS):
THE KEY TO MAKING PROGRESS IN THE INTENSE ACTION PHASE.**

Maximum Muscle Stimulation is directly proportional to the speed **(S)** of each eccentric repetition, that is to say, the contraction part of the repetition and the length of time **(T)** for which one can maintain that speed, rep after rep, without stopping, while engaging the greatest amount of fibers **(F)** while bearing the greatest amount of weight **(W)** for the longest period of time within one's anaerobic capacity. Supplemental to these factors is a person's ability to engage the maximum amount of fibers without over-taxing the nervous system, while still maintaining the greatest amount of overall intensity, stimulated over the least amount of total time spent on any one muscle.

$$T (S + F + W) = MMS$$

Speed of repetitions (S): When I see someone in the gym who is really focused on their muscle stimulation phase, I don't look for and rely on how much weight someone is lifting to gauge whether or not they are stimulating their muscles properly; rather, I watch their speed and repetition fluidity. There is a fine line between moving just the right amount of weight fluidly at a consistent speed (and not stopping until the entire set is complete – which means muscle, not joint, failure.) Excessive movement, a bar that is out of alignment because of too heavy weights, and form that puts the body into disadvantageous positions, are all hallmarks of BAD training. Fluid, consistent repetitions are the hallmarks of good form. You should stop the exercise when your muscles are absolutely exhausted (i.e., at the point of total muscle failure), not at the point where the joint or the nervous system has shut down. While some people will strain themselves trying to lift weights that are too heavy, others err on the other side of the coin. If someone is moving the bar too fast, it is more than likely that the weight is too light for them, and that they are not stimulating the maximum amount of fibers, as is needed to increase muscle mass. For purposes other than warming up, moving an amount of weight that you can lift very quickly is a waste of time.

Conversely, your repetitions should not be moving very slowly, whether in a deliberate fashion or not. If you allow the bar to go slower on the negative half of the repetition, you are not only wasting time, you are also setting the muscle fibers up over a period of time to change in such a way that contractions under heavier weight will become increasingly difficult and eventually impossible. Further, don't let anyone tell you that you will get more stimulation by allowing another person to push up or down upon the bar during the negative part of the rep, this only increases your risk for severe injury, it also decreases your capacity to achieve (MMS) because it decreases the speed of your reps. Remember, near-constant contraction is your goal.

If you are shaking and/or feeling "bogged down" after two or three reps, then the weight you are lifting is too heavy. For bodybuilding purposes, too heavy weights will throw the body into a stressed mode, and will trigger your adrenal glands to release cortisol. An overabundance of cortisol in your system will ultimately lead to nerve damage. Shaking, or a shortened set that occurs because of extremely heavy weight is a sign that you are over-taxing your nervous system (and probably your joints and connective tissue as well). If you do this, you will not be able to stimulate your muscle fibers long enough, or rhythmically enough to achieve good muscle-building results at best, and, at worst, you will begin a process that will lead to serious nerve damage. Your personal safety and longevity should always be your paramount concern.

Finally, if you stop the repetitions for any reason during a set you will lose some of the potential muscle stimulation. It is the building of intensity within the fibers that is the greatest benefit of MMS. Each time you stop, you reduce your intensity, and therefore break up the momentum and perfection of the set. The more intensely you can complete a perfect set, the more stimulation you will gain.

Only use numbers (i.e., counting reps and sets) as a very basic guideline. Focus on your fluidity, and increase the weight over time, but only when you can maintain the same speed and rep range. Imagine your body working like a piston, aim for smooth, disciplined motions bearing heavy weights, continuing until the muscle fails. I will warn you – this is easier said than done!

Time (T): This is a tricky one. I have opted to concern myself with time, rather than numbers of repetitions in a set, for the following reason: notice that the formula is concerned with lifting as it corresponds to time spent within one's anaerobic zone.

Anaerobic capacity, like aerobic capacity, is individual and takes time to build. You will only need to use exact weight calculations to judge set lengths when you are first beginning your program. After you have become familiar with the program, weight and reps will no longer be your major consideration; rather they will become secondary to your quest for form perfection, fluidity, and the pursuit of total muscle failure through MMS. Having said this, anaerobic capacity tends to vary in accordance to an individual's muscle size, ratio of fast to slow-twitch fibers, blood flow, and most importantly, the ability to supply (ATP), the biochemical that stores and uses energy for the muscle to keep moving. [5]

Concern about ATP supply is the chief reason for adding a creatine supplement to your diet. Creatine helps ATP production and uptake, and many double-blind studies have proven its effectiveness in improving results on the bench press, in 40 yard sprints, and squatting. In addition to storing energy, sufficient ATP levels allow the muscles to absorb and utilize water efficiently.

As with any supplement, keep in mind that creatine can have side effects if it is not used properly, and that it is not "the" answer. Most people cannot store more than 10-15 seconds worth of ATP, whether they take supplements or not. This is the fundamental law behind anaerobic, training. If the fibers are being used without oxygen during an intense workout (i.e., MMS), they must rely on ATP for good cellular health and performance during this oxygen-deprived state. ATP infuses the blood with the proper fuel during this anaerobic phase. Because ATP is used very quickly and cannot be stored in mass quantities, no one can lift a lot of weight for a long period of time. We are, after all, primarily aerobic beings. If, however, you can increase your ATP production through supplements and proper nutrition and by working your muscle fibers intensely through regular exercise with increasingly heavy weights, you will eventually be able to lift greater amounts of weight for longer periods of time. Studies have shown that professional weight trainers experience a form of muscle fiber conversion brought about as their amount of weight lifted, increasing through progressively more intense workout sessions. This fiber conversion results in physiologically altered cells, and an increase in all types of fuel and oxygen uptake. If you follow Burke's Law, you will find that your anaerobic capacity will increase, even when you are using heavier weights. You, too, will be altering your muscle fibers the way that professional weight lifters do, at the same time that you are reorganizing your thought processes surrounding lifting and muscle building. This process takes years to complete, but it will happen. Its benefits are worth your effort as you build the body you've always dreamed of, and surpass your previously-held notions about your body's limited capabilities.

It is important to understand and to experiment with anaerobic workouts. For instance, it would not be unheard of for a man to do very heavy leg presses for 25-50 repetitions with only slightly less weight than he could use to complete 20 repetitions.

By working in this intense way, MMS is almost guaranteed, his ATP levels will have been challenged, and an anaerobic threshold has been pushed to its limits. The initial and most difficult stage has been set for maximum muscle growth. You should focus on increasing both strength and this anaerobic capacity so that you can perform moderately heavy sets for as many repetitions as possible. This is especially important for big muscles like the quadriceps, lats, pecs, and so on. Make no bones about it; you are in control of this adaptation, and it takes guts and discipline.

When you can engage the greatest number of fibers **(F)**, while bearing the greatest amount of weight **(W)**, at the fastest speed **(S)** and for the longest period of time **(T)** within your anaerobic capacity, you will have achieved MMS and unlocked the first and most important secret of Burke's Law.

Your Personal Form: Exercises for Each Muscle and Muscle Group

First and foremost, you must develop your training form to perfection. You should find exercises that work for each body-part and stick to them. Don't feel that you must change your routine each time, or every three months, or according to some other schedule that someone of the old paradigm decrees. Really, this is rather foolish, you are an artist, and your body is your canvas. You will work to perfect your form for years, it will take shape in a way that defines you and your style, and in the way that serves you best. It makes no sense to change this perfected form just for the sake of changing it. When you are exercising, your fundamental job is to find your own form and style and stick with it. The equation outlined previously will be easier to understand if you keep this in mind. Find exercises that accommodate your body, your flexibility and bone size will serve as a good predictor for what exercises will be yours. They will be the ones that you feel best performing, and which allow you to control and focus on maintaining a consistent contraction until achieving (MMS). Because you are using your body in a kinetic and biomechanically advantageous way, you will have less chance of injury.

As you seek to perfect your form, your exercise group, work at a certain speed that will allow you to complete all of your repetitions. You will soon determine the speed that allows you to push the maximum amount of weight for enough repetitions to bring your muscle to the point of failure, without stopping or slowing down. This will be another one of the pillars of your success. Your good form and consistency will stimulate the most fibers. Do not be overly concerned with the amount of weight you push, how many sets you complete, or how often you train. Forget about doing your chest on Monday, and legs on Wednesday, and so on. Stop trying to predict how your body is going to react to certain stimuli. You cannot know ahead of time when your body will be at its best. Planning and writing out a workout before you exercise and assuming that you will know how it will affect you and make you feel is foolish. Can you predict what the outcome of rolling a set of dice will be? No, of course not. Therefore, let your body tell you what to do. **Learn the markers, the indicators, the recuperation markers.** You are on a journey that is not dictated by the weekly calendar or a ticking predictable clock. Nothing can stop you now if you realize all this! As you train, you will become aware of many subtleties – how you feel during and after weight work-outs, swimming or other aerobic work, and resting. Only then should you develop your own routine. Listen to your body when it wants to train intensely with weights, or merely wants to take a brisk walk. By allowing yourself this diversity of activity (cross-training), you will learn how your body responds to everything.

Perfecting your form is not as difficult as it may sound. Those who began training under the teachings of the old paradigm, watching Schwarzenegger and the others do things a certain way, assumed that, if it worked well for them, it would work well for everyone. Most people who began training in the late 1970's or 1980's fell under this old paradigm assumption, many, in fact, still do. However, most people fail to consider **three very important points here:** It is a well known fact that many bodybuilders at the ametuer and certainly all of those on the professional level used steroids. (Arnold and many other professional bodybuilders have admitted to using steroids during body buildings' changing era because they were legal, and few if anyone ever questioned their negative effects. Despite the fact that they are now illegal in the US; all professional bodybuilders continue to use steroids, Growth Hormaone, Insulin and many other drugs to enhance their physiques. I would like to see the icon for the great male body look natural, strong and healthy. I believe my body shows this and I believe with the knowledge in this book, your body can look like this also. It takes dedication, hard work and a great visionary to change his body without steroids.) When using anabolic steroids, anyone's body will recover quickly; therefore, the routines of the "old days" were filled with too many sets, not enough cross-training, and not enough days of rest. Furthermore, the routines were developed entirely without consideration for someone over 40 who has diminishing GH and testosterone levels.

Schwarzenegger had a marvelous frame and depth of tissue, so much so that he likely would have been amazing even with no knowledge of the intricacies of bodybuilding. Not everyone has been so physically blessed. This isn't to say that you can't be the next Schwarzenegger, but you will get much more out of Burke's Law than you can out of any outdated Schwarzenegger book – no offense to the "King." I mean no disrespect to Arnold, but these are the facts. You must realize this; you are over 40 and going to gain traction and make progress the way your body will allow you to when you begin this new paradigm.

Often, it is an overachiever who has the greatest ideas, not the greatest champion, for the former must think and experiment more than the latter. Arnold would have won

Mr. Olympia no matter with or without his steroid usage, and would have won it in any decade, for he was genetically gifted and had an uncanny determination that most people cannot muster on one day, let alone for a lifetime.

More on Burke's Law

Let us start by setting some basic rules. Each of these rules must be strictly adhered to, in order to achieve optimum results.

Burke's Fourteen Rules of Motion

1.) Never work out with weights, machines, rubber cables or any other resistance equipment if any muscle is sore. This alone will reduce the number of times you go to the gym down by quite a bit. Conventional wisdom says that it is all right to train your biceps if your calves are sore since it's a different muscle group, but this is fundamentally wrong. If any muscle is sore in any part of your body, especially for those of us over 40, you must not train with weights that day. Rather, on that day, opt to swim, walk, or rest entirely. Heed your body's pattern of ebbing and flowing. Work with it; don't work against it by predetermining your workouts as many people still do.

There are two main reasons for this: first, if you are experiencing soreness, your body's neurological system may have been pushed and has not yet recovered. If you continue to work out, you run the risk of overtaxing your nervous system, regardless of which part of the body you choose to train. Muscle soreness indicates that waste material has not yet been flushed from the body by the lymphatic system. Second, tiny micro-tears within the muscle must have time to heal. These two factors are the main cause for so-called "fitness plateaus." While plateaus do exist, more often, people have simply over-trained, and their body is unable to respond in a positive way to their exercise efforts. You must be sure to account for the natural physical slow-down that occurs as you age. You cannot achieve MMS if you are not ready for it. To be ready for it, your body must be healed and ready to accept change. Based on anecdotal observation, we can conclude that most people go to the gym for weight training far too often. If this is the case, they cannot hope to reach MMS, and therefore are pumping waste-filled blood through already damaged muscles. It would be far better on most days to take a nice brisk walk, go for a swim, or relax than to force yourself through a resistance workout that will only push you backwards.

You should never train with weights unless your body is entirely pain free!

When you were a teenager, your body reacted to stress differently, and even up to age 35 most people can get away with stressing the body before it has fully recovered, but once your reach the age of 40 or 50, it's a whole different ball game. Your goal should be to keep your body balanced, stretched, and growing, and it simply will not grow if you are trying to work in spite of obvious signs of fatigue, such as micro-tears and/or myofascial (muscle tissue) problems. Upon reaching middle age, many people inadvertently take steps backwards by training too much with weights. Knowing when to say no and take a nice walk or pursue some other low-impact activity will save you a lot of pain, time, and effort.

2.) Work out only on days when you feel rested and have had adequate servings of protein, carbohydrates and monounsaturated fats in the previous two to five days. To maintain a successful training program, you must pay attention to the way your body feels, and guarantee that it has had enough of the right kinds of fuel: micronutrients like vitamins and minerals and macronutrients, such as protein, carbohydrates, and fats.

3.) Be sure to consume your proteins, carbohydrates, and fats in a healthy combination. You should eat five or six small meals each day, and each meal should include these three elements.

4.) Don't rely on sports drinks or power bars to give you a last-minute boost before weight training. These are primarily sugar, and as a result will inhibit the release of the vital growth hormone (GH). Without the proper release of GH, you will negate your chances for muscle hypertrophy.

5.) Stretch often. Go swimming, practice yoga, Tai Chi, or some form of passive stretching. If none of the above interests you, take a nice long walk.

You've GOT to stretch, but do it passively!

As your muscles grow, they will shorten, therefore you must take measures to lengthen them in order to prevent injuries. Remember, you cannot stretch a muscle under a load of weight. Do what you can to learn about trigger points, acupressure, acupuncture, and myofascial therapy. Another passive stretching form of exercise is the subtle but effective Feldenkrais Method® [6]. Feldenkrais will show you how much your skeletal frame has changed as a result of weight training stress, and give you a new perspective on how to retrain your autonomic nervous system. The method takes time and patience, but is well worth the effort.

6.) Design a program based on your knowledge of your body, and proceed with confidence. Your methods will work in accordance with those custom-made, personal weight-training sessions that you have been developing, if you follow the advice outlined previously in this book.

7.) Use personal trainers only to learn basic form and how to operate machines in a particular gym. Don't listen too closely to philosophies; most trainers do not think outside the box. Though most are well intentioned, they tend to support the ways of the old paradigm.

8.) Think of muscle growth as both an art and a science. The art comes from devising your own form and workout program. Nothing about your body or your life is entirely predictable; so don't follow a predictable routine. Once you have perfected your form and workout plan (as flexible as it will be), your regiment will become more of a science – one that requires you to listen to your body at all times. Never rely entirely upon your notes to predict when and what you should do before the day actually arrives. Spend six months finding the place and pace for yourself – utilizing all that is available to you. The investment of those six months will pay you back for years to come.

9.) Have a work-out partner help with your weight training only if it is absolutely necessary. I never use one. If you are lifting the correct amount of weight to achieve MMS and still avoid overstraining your muscles, you should be able to manage by yourself. If you cannot, the weight is probably too heavy to do you any good. Forced, or negative reps, do you no good. Rather, you should be working to achieve constant contractions. Prepare yourself both mentally and physically before you walk out onto the gym floor. There is no need to shout or make noise. Allow your energy to flow from within; don't expend unnecessary effort. Building your body can be as much a spiritual event as a physical one. Be within yourself…focus on the goal at hand: maximum muscle stimulation in the shortest amount of time possible. This can really be a wonderful experience.

Make the most of this time with your mind and body in unison.

Focus on the muscles that you are creating. Don't allow self-consciousness to overwhelm you, for fear of who may be watching you. Move beyond the hype of the magazines and the "fraternity" of muscle. This is your one and only chance to live. Consciously inhabiting your own body will make you feel fully alive.

10.) This may sound funny, especially after having described a kind of spiritual bliss attainable by working out in a mindful manner, but if you are interested in someone in the gym, try to wait until the work out is over to make the acquaintance. Don't allow yourself to show off. Romantic interests will come and go many times in your life, but you'll be stuck forever with your wounded body if you aren't focused.

11.) Become a visual, autonomic, physiological, and biomechanical expert when it comes to your body and its subtle messages. Acquaint yourself with every joint, bone, and muscle and be honest to yourself about the genetic hand you have been dealt. You can only compete with yourself. Keep it that way for the peace of all the others who would like to do the same. Show off your body at the beach, not the gym.

12.) Stay away from the scale, and let the mirror and how you feel guide you. As a part of the program you will need to take two body fat percentage tests, but they are purely for calculating daily dietary requirements according to your lean muscle mass. You will test yourself at the beginning of the program, and again six months later, just to make sure that you are on the right track. After the second test, you should be able to look in the mirror and know what needs to be adjusted and how. The mirror doesn't lie.

13.) Don't cheat. If you cheat on yourself, then you aren't really committed to your program. Make the commitment. You have only one body, and will only live this life - make it count. If you are disabled, design a routine that can be done in accordance with your limitations. You will be glad you did. Designing and implementing your routine will be a great challenge, no matter who you are and no matter what physical condition you are in. But remember, it will keep you healthy and you will feel fulfilled and proud of yourself for many years to come, no matter what your ambulatory status is, regardless of the current state of your health – you can help yourself with this program. Never give up on yourself. NEVER! What your body may lack in strength can always be conquered by your strength of spirit. Your strength of spirit will guide you if you listen to yourself closely enough.

14.) Always walk briskly, and do so as often as possible. The neurological, psychological and physiological benefits of brisk walking are impossible to overstate. Walking is probably the single best exercise a person can do. The power of locomotion is a miraculous gift; take advantage of it! Also, swim whenever you can. Swimming allows the muscles and skeleton to elongate, and is also a great form of cardiovascular exercise. Other great choices to round out your training regime are yoga, the Feldenkrais Method®, and Tai Chi.

Chapter Fourteen: Knowledge is Power

Getting to Know Yourself

Though we all have the same number of bones, no two skeletons are identical. Once you clear yourself from serious structural defects, now it is time to get down to brass-tacks. Your muscular-skeletal body has been influenced by everything from heredity and geographic origin to infant nutrition and pre-teenage posture. Together, these factors leave nearly everyone with a "combination frame." You may have thick wrists and skinny knees, or any other number of joint combinations. You need to look at your body and its joints. Assess them, measure them, and understand them. Learn your joints' abilities and limitations, and come to know your skeleton as you may have admired your first car or other significant item in your life.

An intimate awareness of your unique frame is vital for understanding not only your predictable muscle size and strength, but also for determining which exercises should make up your customized fitness routine. Determining the mechanical capacity and potential of each body part is a relatively simple process, and will give you vital information as you devise your fitness plan.

Structural Categories

For many years, kinesiologists, athletes, trainers, and bodybuilders alike have theorized that there are three basic body types: ectomorphs, mesomorphs, and endomorphs. This observation has been based on three fundamental physical characteristics: skeletal structure, the size of existing muscles, and amounts of body fat. Though people occasionally fit neatly into one of these categories, most of us do not. Most of us are a combination of frame, joint and muscle mass that defies specific group-assignment criteria. As you may be able to guess, these "body type" descriptions fall firmly within the realm of the old paradigm. They are terribly unhelpful for most people, and therefore are not a consideration in Burke's Law.

Examine your body as it has been discussed here (and in earlier chapters), take note of what you see and write it down. Three or four months later, reexamine yourself, compare your new findings to the originals, and you will be amazed!

What Each Joint and Limb Should Mean to You

Your arms and legs are, of course, of primary importance when assessing your physical condition because they provide you with locomotive capabilities. They are the catalysts of both your form and function.

Each limb is articulated at three independent, pivotal points. For the arms, this occurs at the wrist, elbow, and at the shoulder, and for the legs, at the ankle, knee, and hip. The wrist and the ankle joints allow your hands and feet to both supinate (turn upward) and pronate (turn downward). There is also a neutral position; for example, the wrist's is a closed fist with the thumb knuckle facing upward. It's important to find the position(s) that give you the best leverage and allows you to exert the greatest amount of force with relative ease. Your hand and forearm strength will dictate much of your upper body potential, as they are the link first in any succession of multi-joint exercises. It is crucial to develop a good grip and find the most advantageous position for completing each exercise.

Tendons attach muscles to bones. The strength of your tendons is primarily based on the length and width of the attaching muscle. The muscle's potential for strength, speed, torque, and velocity correlates to the size of the bone and its tendon. Your potential for muscle shape, size, and speed is 90% genetic. In other words, evolution developed ways for making sure that an individual could not self-destruct as a result of his or her own body weight and/or strength potential. This holds true unless steroids or other muscle-enhancing drugs have supplanted the genetic predisposition.

It is only when you alter your natural hormonal balance with drugs that you can reach beyond the boundaries of your genetic make-up. Steroid abuse is not only biochemically dangerous, it is also physiologically and biomechanically foolish. Tendon and muscle tears are very common among steroid users because the drug allows them to change the systemic form and strength potential of their bodies. Steroids allow the user to make the muscles stronger than the tendons supporting them. Eventually muscles shorten and the tendon will rupture at the site where it attaches to the bone. Knowledge can beat out artificial drugs any day of the week.

You need to focus on the fundamental laws of leverage, form, and Maximum Muscle Stimulation. Be sure that you eat properly, stretch passively, get adequate REM sleep, and develop individual ways to work each muscle group in accordance with Burke's Law. Drugs are not necessary (unless you are going through severe andropause or have hypogonadism – more on these towards the end of the book). The results you will see if you follow these simple steps will prove that steroids are never necessary (and testosterone replacement therapy is only necessary if one/or both of the two above hormonal changes occur).

Top Thirteen Reasons People Do Not Fulfill Their Muscular Potential

1.) Improper assessment of one's kinetic structure

2.) Improper use of advantageous leverage

3.) Misunderstanding of form and functionality

4.) Poor form

5.) Stopping in the middle of sets, cutting down on rhythm and contraction

6.) Improper Intensity

7.) Poor execution of repetitions

8.) Overtraining

9.) Not using other fitness modalities to aid in stretching and keeping the muscle elongated

10.) Becoming bilateral in barbell and machine execution

11.) Improper diet

12.) Inadequate amounts of REM sleep

13.) Hormonal disruption

We have all heard the statement "humans only use only 20% of their brains." Likewise, most people fail to reach even 25% of their fitness potential because they don't know how to identify, and utilize their own strengths, or how to deal with their weaknesses. But, if you pursue a totally natural fitness plan, take nothing but perhaps a basic regimen of vitamins, protein, glutamine, and/or creatine and if you train and eat precisely, you can build a better body than someone taking drugs who is not focused on their training form and nutritional habits. In other words, YES, Burke's Law is as good as taking a muscle-enhancing drug if you follow the program closely and have patience and faith in yourself.

Chapter Fifteen:
Identifying Strengths and Weaknesses

As we have already discussed, in order to fulfill your genetic potential, you must design your own form – that is, designing your own exercises best suited for each muscle or muscle group. You must also find your own range of motion and rhythm according to how an exercise feels and how it may, or may not, be causing muscle hypertrophy. Your form will work in concert with your range of motion and the strengths and weaknesses inherent in your frame. You should start by determining which is your weakest joint affected in each exercise you perform.

General Rules of Motion and Form

There are three very specific points about the correlation between lifting motions and the anatomically correct position that you must maintain when working out. These points are universal, and it is imperative that you proceed in accordance with these rules.

1.) Never put a joint into a disadvantaged, or out of alignment position, this is especially important when performing multi-joint exercises. For example, when working the upper-body, never position a joint in any position other than that of a right angle. You should never perform a bench press with a very close grip, as doing so would put the wrist and hand into unnecessarily stressful positions relative to the upper arm when the weight is lowered. If you were to hold the bench press too closely, your wrist would give out long before your pectoral or triceps muscles – the two groups the press is designed to work – and you would miss out on gaining any possible benefit from the exercise. People look at old-paradigm books that show bodybuilders doing "close grip bench presses." Older books argue that these will work the inner part of the chest; this is anatomically impossible. Your chest will develop according to the way that your genes dictate the location of your pectoral tie-ins and the amount of muscle fiber in that area. Not only is such a promised result anatomically impossible, the exercise itself can prove dangerous. Following the form outlined in the older books will leave your wrists unaligned with your forearms, thus causing a loss of all leverage advantages. Always think of leverage advantage in terms of how equally distributed the weight is across the body at right angles. The only way a chest press can work for anyone is if their forearms are directly in line with their wrists, and the elbows are perpendicular to the machine or your body (depending on whether you use a machine or free weights). Any exercise that puts your wrist, ankle, knee, or elbow in an awkward position will not only cause you to lose your leverage advantage, it will also put the joint in question at risk for injury.

2.) When working the lower body, always keep the knee over the foot, and never put the foot in a position where the ankle has to twist for leverage. When any form of leg-press or squat is being done, keep your knees over your feet, your feet straight, and your thighs relatively straight in relation to your hips – don't let them "bow" out or in too much. It is true that you may be able to create more leverage by placing your feet wider, but if they are too wide, you will run the risk of injuring your knee or ankle.

3.) The stronger the muscle that surrounds the joint, the stronger the joint is. This is the fundamental reason to lift weights: it protects your joints and gives them life-long functionality (provided you don't wear them out by lifting too heavily). So long as you lift moderately and eat properly, your joints will not "wear out." That is to say, there is a point where a weight becomes too heavy and the joint's protective cartilage can either herniate or be worn down by the pressure placed on the attaching bones as they are forced into the joint. Lifting weights should always be done in such a fashion so as to complete a set with minimum of 10-12 smooth lifts without stopping. A good target zone for beginners and intermediates for legs would be 10 to 15 reps per set. More advanced lifters can expect to complete 25-50 reps. Heavy and high-rep sets of each exercise can be achieved once you have become well versed with Burke's Law. You should work to maintain a smooth rhythm. Your reps should have a definite pace to them, and you should complete your set without stopping. Once you stop, the set is over. This is key. If you find yourself shaking during the set, or that the bar is not moving up and down fluidly, you are not in a "groove." The weight is too heavy, which affects your form, and you are taxing your neurological system, ligaments, and tendons more than your muscle tissue.

Always think of these simple rules. Form and groove must be achieved in such a way that you can make your body "remember" without you having to "think" about it, (i.e., work to achieve muscle memory). Once you have muscle memory, don't do anything to change it. You cannot develop your form perfectly if you are shaking during your sets; therefore keep the weight moderate, especially when you are still working to develop your form.

Envision your body and limbs as a group of right angles when you are exercising. For instance, when working the chest muscles, keep your elbows parallel to the bar, or, in some cases, in a straight line with each shoulder, spaced a shoulders' width apart. If you were to move your elbows forward during a bench press, you would be working your triceps muscles more than your pectoral muscles. For instance, when adjusting the height of the seat to do the chest exercise called the "pec-deck," ensure that you sit down and grasp the handles with your elbows up. If you are seated properly, you should see a straight line extending from your hand, to your elbow, shoulder, across your clavicle, over to the next arm, and to your other hand. This line should be maintained throughout the exercise. If your elbows drop, you are not putting all of your resistance on the pectoral muscles. This is a perfect example of how your limbs and joints should be aligned to ensure both MMS and the least possible risk for injury.

Do not move your head when exercising; always look straight ahead. Most body-builders have neck, trapezius, and rhomboid muscle problems because they either turn their heads when exercising, or they "wiggle" their body to force an extra rep. The body and the head should always be still and fixed in one position as the extremities work to pursue a perfect form.

In weight training, your strength capacity can be fundamentally gauged by the strength of your weakest link. Nine times out of ten, your "weakest link" is a joint and the muscles surrounding it. Focus your attention on this area and use the fundamentals of this book to improve the situation.

If an exercise in your workout involves a combination of 3 joints, (such as in the bench, leg, or shoulder press, or a, squat), notice which joint feels the weakest. Chances are that the joint is fine, but that the muscles supporting it are not strong. Here is where Burke's Law should be implemented.

In a multi-joint pulling exercise, such as a pull-up, pull-down, low-row, or barbell-row, it is the length of your limbs and the space of the insertion points of the muscles that will dictate your leverage and strength. In other words, a long arm, with long thick biceps, will develop strength faster than a short arm, when doing pulling exercises. The short arm biceps may reach their potential circumference faster, but long thick biceps will ultimately become bigger, perhaps growing to over 20 inches in circumference, if someone is applying the correct modalities to it. The strength you have available for pulling can be gauged by the length and leverage relative to how long and how thick the attaching tendons and muscles are. On a related note, pushing strength can be gauged by the ability of the muscles surrounding a particular joint to resist collapsing under the weight load, which is too heavy. You should work with weights that allow you to continue pushing throughout a set until muscle failure occurs. When applying Burke's Law, one must remember that everyone's muscles and muscle groups are different. For instance, someone with long arms must "shorten the range of motion" on certain pressing movements so as to lift heavy enough, yet not lose the potential for MMS; this can be done by shortening the range with dumbbells, or on a pressing machine, by adjusting the range. MMS as a mode of weight training is really a matter of inches. Finding your proper place is usually a matter of one notch on the seat or on the range of motion. Just think, only a matter of inches may stand between you and successful MMS, which will improve muscle hypertrophy with each workout and speed the recovery period in your fitness routine.

Evaluating Yourself

Stand in front of a mirror and look at yourself in the buff. The more fiber you have in any one area, or all the muscle areas, the better. You will want to inspect your entire body. Here is an example of how to evaluate two areas:

Examine the width and depth of your pectorals (chest muscles), both major and minor. If both muscles appear "full" up to the clavicles and go down the thorax quite a ways, you have a lot to work with. There are many ways to measure your potential; one of them is to measure the distance between the head of each shoulder (the AC joint) and compare that number to the distance from the lowest part of your pectoral muscles to your belly button. This can tell you a lot, such as how wide your shoulders are relative to the measurement of the difference between the width of your shoulders and the width of your hips and how long your torso is relative to your skeletal structure. The greater the number regarding shoulder girth compared to the width of your hips, the more V-shaped your body will be. Also, measuring the distance between the lowest part of your chest to your belly button will tell you how big your chest can be relative to the abdominal region. The shorter the distance, the more your chest will appear to be appropriately large compared to the upper and lower abdominal area. If these measurements tend to go in the opposite direction, specialty training for deltoid width and specific pectoral exercises will be in order.

Concerning triceps (the muscles running along the back of the upper arm): if all three heads are visible, the longer the triceps; the more potential you have for great muscle development in this area. If you cannot see or find your triceps by feeling the backside of your arm while flexed downward, it is probably due to excess body fat.

Looking now at the lower body, it is important to note the shapeliness of the legs.

The best combination for aesthetic value is to have narrow hips, a vastus lateralus, or the outside of the thigh coming out of the hip-flexor area and sweeping back into just above the knee so as to give an appearance of a large thigh because of the relative size difference between the circumference of the thigh and the circumference of the knee. The same can be said of the calf, from the knee to the ankle.

All of these areas must be honestly assessed so that you can design your program according to these aesthetic proportions, and so that you can implement whichever exercise you feel you have the most biomechanical leverage in. A vision of what you want should always be in your head. The next and sometimes the most important (as demonstrated in earlier chapters) is the back. If no malformations are present; assess your back by using two or three mirrors. Examine it closely. How deep is the crevis on either side of your spine? How wide are the latissimus dorsi muscles? You can feel how low these muscles attach by placing your right hand below your armpit. Squeeze your lats down on your hand, Run your hand down until the muscle tightness stops. Your lat will never attach any lower than this. The old paradigm said that if you had "high" lats, you should do wide pull-ups and pull-downs. Burke's Law simply says, find the most advantageous exercise and blast away. Your lats will grow the way they were intended. You can no more "Lengthen" your lats; than you can "lengthen" your biceps.

Your back is very intricate. Let's take a look at the details of the entire body. The more you can envision and know of your back, the faster you will identify the right exercises for your body.

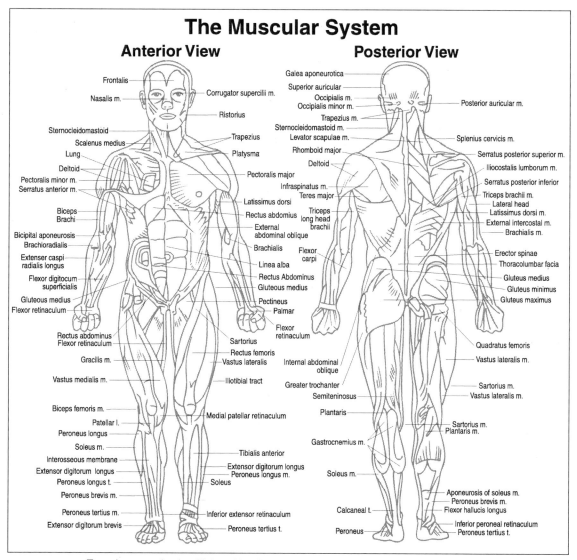

Examine your body. Using this chart, start identifying various muscle groups.

Remember, there are no two bodies exactly alike; therefore no two individuals' workouts should be the same. I cannot emphasize that enough. Everyone who wants maximum muscle size must determine their own strengths and then practice exercises that work well for them, likewise, when it comes to weaknesses, you must find your weak link and address it accordingly. This means to implement a simple seat adjustment, shortening the stroke, or the stretch. It may mean using dumbbells instead of a bar. It may mean that you use cables, or rubber cables for a time to get at weak area in the middle of your back. You will find a way, but you must clear your head of what has been said in the past concerning "the right way and the wrong way."

Don't be overly concerned about your range of motion matching a predetermined model by contemporary thinking. You will start with your own natural range of motion, and work from there – this is where your potential strength lies. This is the key to maximal repetitive stimulation with minimal loss of leverage. You must first find the place where leverage is lost in every movement, when your muscles are under a moderate to heavy load. Then you must identify the precise moment in the movement when the muscles you are working are most engaged before the "weak link" is activated and you lose leverage, and will not be able to achieve MMS. By identifying this point, you can use it as a reference in determining where your greatest strength relative to "range of motion" is in each exercise.

Examples to Visualize

Let's start with a well-known pushing movement, the bench press, and use it to examine two extreme biomechanical examples of leverage – or the lack thereof. First, picture the standard "full range of motion" for someone on a bench press. Imagine the person performing the press has a large rib-cage girth, relatively short arms, wide shoulders, and pectorals that attach low on the rib cage and high on the clavicles. Biomechanically, this person is "built" for the bench, and will therefore be able to master the exercise with ease. The thick rib cage shortens the stroke of the repetition automatically if you assume that "all-the-way-down" means touching the bar to the chest. With this bit of information alone, we can see that the "standard range of motion" cannot be "standard" at all, since this distance is unique to every body. Likewise, the shorter the arms, the shorter the distance the weight must travel from the bottom point to arm extension. Already, this person has two huge structural advantages when thinking of the bench press. Now, let's say that he also has wide shoulders, a leverage-gaining advantage. His wide shoulders allow him extra comfort and a wider grip on the bar, all achieved without "pinching" the arms out too far, which can cause rotator cuff problems. A person with narrow shoulders can use a wider grip to shorten the stroke, but there is a point of diminishing returns where his leverage will be lost as his hand spacing moves further away from his natural shoulder width. Further, involvement of the pectoral muscles also compromises wrist strength in relation to the wider grip. With this example, we can see that our first character, with his wide shoulders and full rib cage will have an easy time with the bench press, but we can also see that there really is no "standard" for range of motion – his genetic gifts that make the press easy for him to have a much shorter range of motion than our other example, the man with the narrower shoulders. Here is where genetics appear to rule; however, by applying Burke's Law, the disadvantaged person may indeed be able to overcome his weakness.

We can attribute our first subject's great leverage advantage to his pectoral muscles, which are attached low on the rib cage – reaching thickly all the way to the clavicles. Obviously, he has more muscle fiber with which to work. The more fiber involved, the more efficiently weight can be pushed, and the greater potential there is for muscle development. A perfect example of someone who had wide shoulders and low pectoral tie-ins with enormous muscle mass is Arnold Schwarzenegger. Ironically, Schwarzenegger's weakest upper body muscles were triceps. They were weak because he had been so genetically gifted in terms of his enormous amount of pectoral tissue and wide shoulder girth that each time he bench pressed (which he did a lot), almost all of his pushing power was exerted by his pectoral muscles. As a result, his triceps were rarely worked when he used heavy weights in pressing movements.

If you see someone with long arms and wide shoulders but "high-pecs," it is more than likely that this person will have shallow pectorals and big, thick triceps. Why? Because during multi-joint pressing (such as the bench press) this person's genetics have led him to use his triceps more than his chest during pushing movements. Had either of these men been following Burke's Law, they would have been able to bring their weak points up to par. Keep in mind; genetics plays a large role in the development of any muscle.

Each of the factors cited in our first example contributes to a multiplication of advantages, all of which allow our subject to become stronger and larger by working within a standard form. Further, as his pectoral muscles grow larger, his stroke (range) will be further reduced, thus increasing his natural leverage even more. Because of his multiple advantages and the multiplication of advantages, his strength will increase exponentially as he continues to exercise.

Even if you weren't genetically blessed with multiple advantages, there are ways to gain these advantages by adjusting your range of motion with dumbbells or by shortening the range on a machine. Remember, only one or two inches lies between success and total failure. Don't choose someone else's idea of where that critical inch should be.

Using Burke's Law to Your Greatest Potential

Imagine a person of relatively the same height and weight as our first example, but one with a shallow rib cage, long arms, narrow shoulders and high pectoral tie-ins. He has virtually no upper pectoral fiber to work with. If he tries to employ the standard "full range of motion" for this exercise, then, he will have a great deal of difficulty. It is easy to imagine this person being "buried" under a weight that our first subject could have pressed 20 times with ease. If you have ever watched a person built in this way performing free-weight bench presses, you probably saw someone struggling with the weight, doing individual reps all the way up and down, all in a vain attempt to build his upper body. This person has a multiplication of disadvantages, each of which contribute to and magnify the others, resulting in a slow process of failure at best, and horrible injury at worst. Over time, his pursuit of the so-called "standard full range of motion," will likely lead to injury. In the process, he will have seen very little progress in his quest for improved strength and muscle size. It is the "full-range" of motion itself that is the cause of difficulty for those with a genetically disadvantaged upper body, when performing this exercise.

Luckily, there is a happy medium between using enough weight to stimulate the pectorals while successfully performing a range within the reps so that changes in range will help fatigue the muscle before the "weak link" gives out. The answer in this case is in short dumbbell strokes, or adjusting arm range on the chest-pressing machine. The body responds to targeted muscle stimulation; it has no clue what a "full range of motion" is or is not. Changing just one inch so as to allow you to contract the muscles in rhythmic, fluid style makes all the difference in the world.

Of course, these are two extreme examples, and generally speaking few people are either. For those who fall into the weak-pushing disadvantage situation, have no fear, there are many more components of Burke's Law that are designed to help you make the most of your genetic potential.

These "range of motion" reps and sets developed many years ago by the founding fathers of bodybuilding are logical on paper and in person for those who it works well for. But, what if it doesn't work for you? Do you struggle and be plagued by injuries? Or, do you come up with a creative answer. For instance, if your bench press is weak and dumbbells don't help, consider doing decline bench presses because this will shorten the "range" and for those of you with big shoulders and weak pecs; it will take the shoulders out of the set. This is creative thinking. This is real life, with real variables that every body has. Today our challenge is to rewrite the book of form and function to maximize each person's potential, without injury, without frustration, and without failure.

In the past, it was believed that shortening reps would cause you to become "muscle-bound." This was based on the notion that a shortened range would result in shortened, improperly stimulated muscles, but this is a huge fallacy. If it were true, a carpenter who hammers nails all day would find that his hammering arm is locked into a range of motion of only 45 to 60 degrees, and he would not be able to extend or contract his biceps muscle fully. We now know that the muscles shorten in weight training no mater what the range. This is why a stretching program must be used in addition to weight training. This is also why it is logical to have your own "range of motion according to your body; muscle group per muscle group."

Often times a pushing muscle will respond better when the range is shorter because you can increase rhythm and intensity, and maintain a continuous, pulsating tension; contracting the muscle quicker and more often. This is the recipe for greater contraction consistency. This can often be achieved most effectively with dumbbells or with variable-range weight machines. By shortening the range of motion, you can use more weight, put less pressure on weaker joints, and achieve form and function with proper intensity. Also, this method will allow for a constant engagement of muscle fibers, thereby achieving the all-important state of MMS. If you are older and/or injured, using rubber cables may be the ideal apparatus for you. Remember, these shortening ranges in exercises are for pushing muscles only; it just so happens that bodybuilding is easier when the range of motion in pressing movements is shorter. While this applies only to "pushing" motions, Burke's Law sets out to reinvent the laws of bodybuilding, so I devised exercises for pulling motions as well.

By examining each muscle system in your body, you will become conscious not only of how the body functions during weight and fitness training, but also of how these systems integrate with and support one another. This understanding will lead you to perfect form for each of the exercises that you design in range, repetition, intensity, constant contraction and leverage advantage. The load has been lifted, so you no longer have to feel confused about so many theories. THIS IS THE ONLY THEORY THAT IS PROVEN AND WILL WORK FOR EVERYONE.

Ideal exercises for each area of the body, in accordance with body structure awareness, are the keys to your total body success.

The following muscle groups and alternative exercises are given to give you an example as to how to go about making up your own exercises for each of your body parts. This is a shortened list of exercises and I have added graphics to clear the pathway for a visual understanding. Remember, for every muscle group, there will be a weakness in everyone; however, the ideology here is to maximize your potential in all areas.

Trapezius

If your shoulders are wide and straight, your traps will most likely respond to two or three major exercises.

1.) Barbell shrugs: This motion should be straight up and down with no rolling forward using the scapula (shoulder blade) muscles, or pulling too far back. If you have wide shoulders, these exercises involve shoulders, but isolating the traps should be easily applied. For those of you with narrower shoulders, you will have to be more creative in your exercise choices.

2.) Upright rows: These should be done in a deliberately up and down fashion. Squeeze just beneath your chin and nothing more but fluid determined reps.

3.) Side lateral raises can be performed with dumbbells while sitting on a bench. You should squeeze the traps together at the top of the motion for help in developing this area.

These exercises should be done in a full range both up and down with no shoulder rolling or positioning the shoulders so that the scapula is turned up, in the archetypal "most muscular" pose. With this body shape, you should have a fairly easy time developing your traps and shoulders, especially if they are naturally wide and relatively square.

If your shoulders are more rounded and hang slightly to moderately forward, both your traps and posture will respond to taking a pair of moderately light dumbbells and shrugging them up and back as far as possible, contracting the traps and rear deltoids and moving your scapulas inward. Be careful not to use your biceps and pull the weight up with their assistance. The arms should be straight and locked at all times when performing this exercise. This will make your shoulders move back and build your traps in such a way as to help with your posture. Drooping, rounded shoulders are not good and can lead to any number of problems. Be certain, however, that you don't make the situation worse with weight training. Always pull up and back; never roll your scapulas forward by applying pressure in an already poor postural alignment. Rounded, sloping shoulders need to be worked back at all times. Even when walking you should make a conscious effort to keep your shoulders back, your head up as far as possible, held straight, yet tilted slightly down.

This body's overall shape can also benefit from upright rows, performed with a bar attached to a floor pulley and cable. You should stand approximately 2-3 feet from the cable's attachment site, and pull the bar toward your chin while squeezing the shoulders back. You should not let the weight pull your shoulders all the way forward, nor should you ever let the bar go all the way down (meaning, let your arms relax, a motion which would tend to pull the shoulder forward). Aim to go half to three quarters of the way down and right back up again, remembering to keep the elbows slightly pointed up and shoulders pushing the traps together and back. Always pull your shoulders back if they tend to be rounded and droop forward. The objective here is to get your traps to respond because the shoulders are being brought back. Work to complete failure, for 15-20 reps on these exercises. Work non-stop and with as heavy a weight as you can handle while keeping your neck muscles relaxed.

Shoulders

Many people do all sorts of strange exercises for their shoulders, like the so-called "Arnold-press" that incorporates a host of irrelevant movement. This, and a whole host of other exercises that incorporate far too many muscles to truly isolate the deltoids, is not only generally ineffective, it also has the potential for causing real harm. For any type of body that is free of injury, pressing straight up and down is the best way to build the shoulders. Your shoulders' shape, like almost every other part of your body, is genetically predetermined, we must remember this. Therefore, to build your shoulders beyond their natural capacity, you should aim to press as heavy a weight as possible for as many reps as possible, without pause. When I say "heavy as possible," this means that you have to still stick to the rules of smooth rhythmic non-stop reps. Evolution developed our shoulders to assist in pushing straight over-head, and it is in the genetic coding of your makeup that will determine what they "look like" when they are fully developed. Therefore, there is no need to try to "shape" shoulders with specific exercises, because your shoulder shape will always be governed by the bounds of your genetics.

To develop your shoulders to their fullest potential, you must determine where your greatest leverage is in relation to the pressing motion. Here are a few tips to keep in mind when thinking about shoulder leverage:

1.) Be sure that the bench that you are pressing from isn't too low or too high. The lower the bench, the higher your knees will be in relation to your hips, thus putting yourself at a huge leverage disadvantage. The same is true for the opposite situation; if the bench is too high you will have no stability. Remember, the seat for any pressing movement, including bench presses, should place your thighs and knees even with your hips. The lower part of your leg should be at a perfect right angle with your thigh, and your feet should rest flat on the floor. Proper positioning of the entire body will make up to a 20% difference in not only your power but also in the control you have over the weights. Take the time to find the right sitting position before you begin. Just think "parallel and 90 degrees" with respect to all pressing motions with arms and legs.

2.) Before pressing, always be sure to warm up your biceps, so that you will have a little "cushion" to assist in your pressing motions. You might also want to warm up your forearms a bit too, as they are important for pressing success, especially if you are using dumbbells. Warmed up muscles will allow you to squeeze the bar better. The more control you have over every aspect of the exercise, the better your results will be, it's that simple. Pumping up muscles such as the biceps and forearms are worth at least 15% extra intensity because the pumped biceps will act as a cushion at the bottom of the rep; and, as said previously, the forearm is critical in bar, handle, or dumbbell control.

If you have wide shoulders, you will do much better with a free-weight bar. People with medium to narrow shoulders do best with dumbbells, and/or seated shoulder pressing machines that allow for range adjustment. For whichever apparatus you choose to work with, move it straight up and down and do not stop until you are fatigued. Don't allow yourself any funny "arching" motions, or to move or rotate the dumbbells. The palms of your hands should stay facing away from your body, and you should maintain the pressing exercise until achieving fatigue and no more. Make sure the seat is set at the perfect angle for you and take care not to lock your joints for even a single rep. Push the weight up almost to a locking position, and then bring it down again. Work to be able to handle heavier weights for more reps. I cannot stress this enough. You must increase both weights and total reps. It does you no good to increase weights but only mange five reps. Minor adjustments, such as seat location, foot placement, how square your body is with the weight in your hands, and how can you increase weight and reps without losing form, speed, or repetitive intensity will all bring you to a place where you can achieve your maximum potential. Good pressing is an art and you must work on your form very hard before advancing to heavier weights. Use as few muscles as you can, in order to isolate the muscles you are working with a more difficult modality. Isolation, concentration, contraction, intensity, and MMS will lead you to muscle hypertrophy.

Let's take a moment now to think about barbells versus dumbbells. Many people choose to work primarily with dumbbells. If you, too, make this choice, it would behoove you to work on your forearms twice weekly, in order to strengthen them. This conditioning should be separate from the light biceps and forearms pumping you do before pressing. The stronger your forearms are, the more capable you will become at handling heavy dumbbells. The stronger your grip, the less you need to concern yourself with balance, and the more you can focus on building your shoulder muscles. Of course, this advice does not only apply to shoulder work, but generally for all exercises that involve the use of your hands. By making your grip as firm as possible, your results will be that much greater.

Bent Over Side Laterals: This is the single best specialty exercise for the rear deltoids of the shoulders. In addition to the bent over position, this exercise can also be done sitting facing a pec-deck and pulling the handles back as far as possible to squeeze the rear deltoids and rhomboids together. This can also be done by using dumbbells which can give almost anyone an overall better result. To perform this exercise, keep your back flat, knees slightly bent and raise the dumbbells as far out and up as possible, with your elbow slightly bent so as not to injure the elbow joint. Try to establish a nice rhythm, and squeeze your rear deltoids and the center of your back together as much as possible. As a rule, you should complete at least 12-15 reps and really pump them out. Using a moderate weight is key here because, as you know by now, form is everything. Working your back on "shoulder day" is not the way to achieve good results, so be sure that you isolate your rear deltoids and really get them burning. Burning isn't necessarily a feeling you want with all muscles, but when you isolate small muscles, and push out the reps, a burn will probably follow.

Chest

With the exception of the arms, the chest is the body part that most people work on the hardest. It is, after all, the focal point of the front of the body for both men and women. Ultra-firm abdominals may have become very trendy in recent years, but making your abs show is largely a matter of diet. Getting the chest to grow can be a relatively easy task for some, but for others it is an ongoing frustration. If you are among the many who do have trouble with this area, the following tricks will prove particularly useful.

Bench Press: This is potentially a very dangerous exercise, no matter how easy it may seem to you. Simply put, it places a huge strain on the shoulder joints, especially the rotator cuffs, and, for some, elbow bone spurs can occur. Also, everyone tends to be stronger on one side than the other; therefore we tend to force the strong side to bear the brunt of the weight when performing this exercise, while the other arm is struggling to balance and stabilize the weight on a free weight bar. Another problem that arises from this disproportionate sharing of the workload is the stress it places on the nervous system. The risk for developing rotator cuff problems, chronic pain, and a myriad of injuries is simply too high with this exercise; unless you are absolutely certain that your body is perfectly, bio-mechanically suited to execute this exercise without any negative pain at all. If you feel you must bench press, the best advice is to do so very rarely, and work only with dumbbells of a moderate weight for 10 or more repetitions. By using dumbbells, you will use your muscles symmetrically; whereas barbells tend to build bilateral strength.

When some people use a barbell for shoulder or chest presses, they can easily inadvertently pinch their AC (acromioclavicular) joint. This happens when the bar is used in a disproportionate way, and thus causes havoc upon the entire upper trap, shoulder and neck area. If this happens repeatedly, you run the very real risk of tearing your assessory nerve. Never tell yourself that you can "work through" pain. This is a major mistake. If you work through pain in this area, your shoulder will eventually become inflamed to the point where your trapezius, sternocleidomastoid and other muscles in the neck may go into a severe spasm and lock. The assessory nerve, which runs from the neck (at about C-2 on the spine) to the shoulder, down the latissimus (side of back) muscles and up again to the trapezius muscles at the base of the skull. These muscles can become so inflamed from constant work and pinching of the AC joints, often the muscles will go into spasm and cause assessory and/or the long thoracic nerves can become stretched or ruptured. This then can severely, if not permanently be damaging to your fitness and weight lifting life. Heavy bench-pressing with a bar can cause lots of inconceivable damage. Permanent rotator cuff and AC joint problems are so common it is only the severe nerve damage injuries that even raise an eyebrow at the orthopedics office. Shoulder replacements are all very common conditions among weightlifters now. When it comes to working the chest, unless you have never experienced an injury in your shoulder, use dumbbells, cable crossovers, or some sort of weight machine designed for the chest, such as a "pec-deck" or a plate-loaded pressing machine, and use them in moderation!!! These apparatuses allow for freedom of movement that a bar does not, and will therefore help you to work your chest muscles without fear of serious injury.

If you are currently doing bench presses and are not experiencing any shoulder problems, chances are that, if you use moderate weight and good form, you will be OK. But for those of you who have experienced any shoulder pain or injuries, do not perform any pressing movements with a bar or a Smith Machine. These are simply too restrictive for your body type, and at some point their restrictions will cause either a severe rotator cuff problem, or perhaps even a ruptured or torn nerve.

As mentioned before, preparing to press by warming up the biceps and forearms can help you with your dumbbell pressing routine. Make sure that your legs are in the right position in relation to your body, the bench, and floor, as they will be able to give you added leverage. Never put your feet up on the bench. Though folk wisdom once held that putting one's feet up while bench pressing puts more emphasis on the chest, this is not true. All it really does is destabilize your body and make you look like a fool.

Another important component of the chest press puzzle is the positioning of your lumbar spine area. You should keep this area slightly arched away from the bench and your chest slightly up in the air while performing a press. Maintain this position for the entire set, and take care only to a move your arms and shoulders up and down in a smooth, pumping motion. Your hand spacing, whether you are using a bar or dumbbells, is very important. Keep your hands no more than one or two inches beyond the width of your shoulders. If you place them further apart, you will be putting your wrists in a disadvantaged position and also will be pinching your rotator cuff.

Remember, keep your chest up, pump only the chest, and do rep after rep, without stopping until you reach failure. An ideal set would involve 8-12 reps but as with the other exercises discussed here, you must identify your weak spot, and bring the dumb-bells down no further than necessary before pushing them back up again. There is a happy medium between bringing the dumbbells down all the way, which for some is too far, touching your shoulders, and finding that place just above the shoulders and being able to blast back up like a piston. If you have an exercise that you really feel good performing, such as a decline dumbbell press, then do four or five hard-fought sets and one finishing exercise and call it a day. The object is to stimulate the greatest amount of fibers in the shortest period of time (MMS). If you can really use a heavy load and build your anaerobic capacity, you may find yourself doing only three or four sets for your chest, but, you will not be able to do this until you are at the point where you know exactly what it takes to stimulate just enough so that the fibers will repair in time for your next workout. You must work toward knowing how much is enough, how much is too much, and how intense your training must be, for these are the factors that will influence not only your potential recovery time, but also your ability to increase your anaerobic capacity under a heavy load and therefore achieve the greatest stimulation and maximize your potential for hypertrophy. All of this, after you have found the perfect exercise, your perfect range of motion and perfect form and concentration for each and every individual muscle and muscle group.

Triceps

For most people, the key to developing the most fibers possible within their triceps is to ensure that they make a tight lockout with each rep. This is one of only a few muscle groups for which I make this recommendation. Because of the way the triceps work, and because of their three attachment points, the harder you can squeeze them under the heaviest possible load, rep after rep until failure, the more they will be stimulated to their maximum potential. So, when choosing a triceps exercise, choose one that you feel gives you the most leverage and allows you to lift the most weight, while maintaining the most stable bodily form (position) possible. Two exercises that I find helpful are the triceps pushdowns and overhead extensions.

When performing a triceps pushdown, try to use as much weight as you can, for 12-20 reps, making certain to lock each one out at the bottom for just a split second. Do not hold the lock for long. Overhead extensions are best performed with a straight bar, hitched to a cable behind the head. This will result in the weight forcing a total collapse of the triceps onto the biceps. To push the bar out, you should be bent over slightly, with the cable handle almost in front of your face at extension. This position will allow you to feel every fiber in your triceps contraction. You should allow the triceps to collapse fully, and then push outward over your head until the triceps are fully extended and contracted. This works for everyone because of the position and function of the triceps.

Personally, I prefer these two triceps exercises to all others. I never deviate from them, and my triceps are very well developed. Having said that, however, I must note that I have worked on them for thirty years to achieve and maintain their condition. This book should not influence you to think that only those particular exercises are going to be the "right" ones, or the only exercises for you; you must determine that for yourself. Once you do find the exercises that make you feel best in terms of your strength, stability, and form, stick with those exercises! Do not change.

Back

The back is a very complex group of muscles. Because you cannot see your back while you are working out, it is a good idea to look at the anatomical chart on page 79 and familiarize yourself with the area. You will be amazed at how complex and diverse the muscle shapes are, and by how many directions the muscles crisscross all over the back.

Before going any further, we must talk about width. One of the key features that distinguishes bodybuilders from contact sports participants, or other weight-trained athletes, is the width of their backs. Many people will tell you that the first time they saw someone with big lats, they could hardly believe that such a thing was possible. It is impressive; there is no doubt about it.

The latissimus dorsi (lats), infraspinatus, and the teres major muscles comprise the outer edges of the muscles that give width to the upper back. There are many ways to build these muscles, but uppermost on most lists, and in the realm of Burke's Law, is pull-ups. A pull-up is to lat width what a curl is to biceps circumference. There is no question, no matter what your shape, pull-ups should be included in your routine. But how should they be done?

For most people, the conventional wisdom of the old paradigm remains their mantra: the further out (or apart) you hold your hands, the further out your "point of attack on the lat muscle will be." While this is plausible, it is not necessarily true, as many kinesiologists and even Mike Mentzer have discovered. Instead, always combine wide-grip overhand pull-ups with narrow-grip underhand pull downs. Do them one right after another in "super-set" fashion. The rationale behind this method is that all three of these muscles are attached and designed to move in different directions, each with differing results. Thus, a big "stretch" could actually come from a narrow grip, and a wide grip will make certain muscles contract at the bottom, or at the starting point. When these two exercises are combined, you will be able to exhaust the lats, infraspinatus, and teres major muscles very quickly. Once you have gotten to the point where you can do no more pull-ups, try hanging from the bar and pulling with your lats, to move your torso three or four inches up and slightly forward without pulling with your arms. This is a wonderful way to finish off a back workout. When it comes to lats, the longer you can hang there and move, the better. So, try to complete twelve solid pull ups, taking care to arch the spine and contracting the back at the top of each rep, then move immediately to the pull-down machine, using a close-grip and straight bar, for twelve more. Then do shoulder-width overhand pull-ups on the bar until you cannot move any more. After two or three rounds of this, you will have done everything possible to increase the width of your back. I recommend using a straight bar, but you may find V-bar pull-ups more effective for your body. Or, you may find that underhand grips work better for you than overhand ones. Again, this is fine. This is why you must look at your frame, come to understand how these muscles work, and then determine how you are going to activate the greatest amount of fibers in the shortest amount of time. One side note – while speed is certainly something to concern yourself with, be sure to rest for a minute or two after each set to allow your ATP to build back up, otherwise you will be working aerobically, not anaerobically, and will lose out on muscle-growth potential. You will know when it is time to rest and time to go as you become more acquainted with this style of training. And keep in mind; it takes many years to get your anaerobic capacity to a point where you can really train for extended periods of time with moderately heavy weights.

You must focus on understanding your skeletal structure, its attaching muscles, and tendons to find the right combination of exercises for you. Once you have accomplished this, you will begin to see where your natural advantages and disadvantages lie. Always work in accordance with your natural advantages, because, as we have already discussed, your muscles will ultimately be shaped by your unalterable genetic coding. Stimulate them however you can, and in time, they will grow to fullest potential and shape.

In addition to back width, you need to consider back thickness. To increase thickness, you will rely mainly on intense muscle contractions. Perhaps the most effective exercises for improving back thickness are low pulley rows, done with a full stretch and deep contractions. Take care to pull the bar back toward your stomach, and contract as many muscles in the center of your back as possible. There are many weight machines available to help achieve this deep contraction in the back muscles; try them all before finalizing your routine. One thing to consider is using these machines for "crunching" the muscles together, without ever extending your back muscles completely.

Barbell rows are excellent exercises for addressing thickness, as are dead-lifts. Though these moves are staples for back thickness, most people over 40 should exercise caution when performing them. If done improperly, you run the risk of herniating a disc or causing other severe lower back problems. If you have never done these exercises, or haven't for many years, don't start now. You can always build your erectus spinae muscles (those that straighten the torso from a bent position) by doing Hyperextensions.

Hyperextensions are the opposite of sit-ups. Hyperextensions are performed on a special bench that places you facedown towards the floor, your hips at the edge of the Hyp-bench – your feet should be hooked beneath two rolling rubber pads to allow you to lower your upper body, face down, toward the floor until your upper body is 90 degrees to your legs.

Hyperextensions extend and contract your lower back, and are best executed by putting your hands behind your head and forcing all of your back muscles to contract toward the ceiling. Hyperextensions are an ideal "finishing" exercise. If you want to, raise your body up and slightly back – arching the lumbar area. If you find this easy, you can put a weight behind your head, 10-20 pounds is sufficient, but be sure to work up even to this seemingly light weight. Most people do not need weight.

There are many other very valid back exercises, such as T-bar rows, barbell rows, and one-armed rows, and on and on the list goes. As usual, determine which ones, or which machines, you really feel powerful using and pursue them to their fullest. You only need to use two or three for a total of 10-12 sets for your entire back, but you should be sure to remember to work towards increasing intensity and decreasing your number of sets. Once you are very comfortable with the exercises and their affect on your body, you should be able to do three to five total sets for the entire back. Remember, this is what you are working toward, to be able to achieve MMS in an entire area of muscles in a few sets; however, this takes a lot of mental and physical work. Work slowly, and in time you will be able to achieve MMS in increasingly short periods of time.

Biceps

After the chest, biceps are the muscles that people seem to be the most impressed by. But, let me remind you, never ask someone with great biceps how they got them so big. No matter what answer you receive, it will not help you. You need to determine what regimen is best for you, not copy what worked for someone else. Chances are, a person with phenomenal biceps also has big wrists, ulna, and radius bones, that their biceps attach low on their arms, and that they had a naturally thick cross-section of muscle fibers to work with. If you already have great biceps, you know this first-hand. If you haven't been blessed with naturally great biceps, this is the point where true imagination and your work to develop your body as a piece of art comes into play. The biceps are one muscle group where, with enough hard work, you can hope to outpace your genetic predisposition. By working with your wrists and hands facing upwards you can develop a better lifting form, and thus achieve great "peaked" muscle growth.

Without a doubt, the location where your biceps attaches to the ulna bone (how long your biceps tendon and muscles are) and your fiber thickness in that area will determine how big the biceps will naturally be; however, there are a few creative ways to maximize an otherwise weak body part.

The old paradigm approach says that, if you have high attachments on the biceps bottom attaching point, you should do a lot of Scott curls (also known as "preacher curls") because they will "lengthen" the tendon (and thus the muscle). This is pure rubbish. You cannot change a tendon's attachment point, nor lengthen your biceps tendon. Attachment points are fixed at birth, and no matter which exercises you choose, you cannot change them. Hyperextending your arm in an attempt to lengthen the tendon insertion point will only leave you with a ruptured biceps tendon.

Isolation is the key to building your biceps. Even though isolation is required for any sort of muscle building, the biceps, especially those that attach high and have thin cross-fibers, is of the utmost importance. People with weak biceps tend to overcompensate during arm exercises by utilizing their shoulders (which, ironically, but usually are quite good). So, one of your first considerations should be to get your shoulders out of the exercise. An ideal exercise for achieving this is the concentration dumbbell curl, performed with your arm hanging down while you support your slightly bent-over body with your other arm placed on your knee. You should be bent over with your elbow just slightly forward of the shoulder and the weight must be raised and lowered without moving the upper arm or shoulder at all. Begin with a moderately light weight, so that you can ensure your form is perfect. Concentrate on your form to make certain that the shoulder is entirely out of the picture; this may take months, because muscle memory is very strong, but you will not be disappointed. The more often and perfectly you can do this, the better your biceps will look. (This motion is known as "supinating:" raising the dumbbell and turning the right wrist clockwise as far as possible at the end of the repetition.) At the beginning of the exercise, your wrist should be in a neutral position, with your arm hanging down, the weight in your hand, and your wrist aligned with it. The object of this "concentration" curl is to pull the biceps up and rotate your wrist clockwise as hard as possible while flexing your biceps and keeping all of your other muscles out of use for the curl. This must be practiced over and over correctly to change the shape of your biceps; however, once you find your groove and weight, you will be amazed at how massive and peaked they can become. (The left wrist would be turned counter-clockwise.)

Standing curls are another good exercise for building the biceps. Many people practice standing curls, but often their form is either too rigid, or too loose (they swing their bodies too much). If you already have good biceps and standing curls are already a staple of your routine, keep doing them. To build the muscles even more, simply add a small amount of movement, so that you can add a bit of extra weight. A big swing is nothing more than a reverse-hand clean (as in the Olympic lift, the "clean and jerk"). If your standing curls are performed with good form, you will be able to build some "softballs" in no time.

Scott curls (aka, preacher curls) are one of the best exercises for biceps, and can be done much in the same fashion as forearm work. Start by doing 8-10 reps, then pull them up higher and higher, each time dropping the forearm less, until you are only moving the dumbbell, bar, or grip on the machine up and down an inch or so, as if you were trying to crack a walnut between your biceps and forearm. Curl up and up for maybe a minute after the first part of the set is finished. This will be a tremendous help to you in building your biceps.

Forearms

According to Burke's Law, there is only one way to work the forearms. You should grasp a moderately heavy barbell, rest it on your thighs while seated, squeeze as tightly as you can, and then lower it parallel to the floor, so that the hand, wrist, and forearm are all in a straight line. With each rep, bring the barbell up higher using only your forearms to move the wrist, until you are barely moving it up and down at all. By the end of the set, and for 30 seconds or more afterward, you should only be moving and squeezing the bar a half inch, always trying to pull it closer and closer to your elbow, or ulna-flexor, the belly of the forearm. If you must, go up on your tiptoes and remain there until failure of your forearms. Squeeze and move the barbell towards your forearms – not towards the floor. Do this until you can no longer stand the pain, then put the bar down and wait 20 seconds, then repeat the process again. Do this twice a week, occasionally adding some Zotman curls, and your forearms should respond well.

Waist

Perhaps 40% of the questions I am asked about fitness have to do with abdominal work and how to obtain a "six-pack." Abs themselves are not usually the real problem, rather it is the fat covering them that should be addressed. You only need to work your abs a little, maybe twice a week. Leg raises, either done while hanging from a pull-up bar, or lying supine and holding onto something above your head are an ideal exercise for abdominal conditioning. You only need to do a few sets of each, and add a few crunches, then, let your diet do the rest of the work. Getting ones abdominal muscles to show through the skin is almost entirely dependent upon the amount of one's body fat. It's that simple. The nutrition and longevity chapters of this book will provide you the answers you need to have better abs.

Legs

For people over 40 who do not use performance-enhancing drugs, the legs are one of the most difficult parts of the body to develop without the gift of big, shapely thighs and calves. No matter what your age, the amount of stimulation required to build the thighs and calves is quite high, therefore figuring out the right exercises and then achieving measurable success with them are two totally different things. Nothing is impossible, though, so you can make progress, no matter what your genetics say.

Squats are a good exercise for developing the leg muscles. If you have been squatting for some time and are pleased with your results, don't change a thing. If, however, you haven't seen the response you'd like, keep squatting, but keep the following in mind:

1.) If you are already a "seasoned squatter," perform one warm-up set, one set at 65% for 12 reps, then a final set at 75% of as many as you can possibly do until complete failure. Set the bar so that you can use a "stripping method" with your weights. Work to reach your upper weight threshold, where you cannot complete any more reps, then strip 20% of the weight, and do as many more reps as possible. Follow this reduction pattern until you are at the point of fatigue, then put the bar down and count to 30. Pick the bar up again, taking it from the squat rack and resting it just below your neck on your traps. Then, do as many reps as possible with whatever weight remains on the bar.

If you have never squatted before, but would like to try, follow this method. Master your form by using just the bar, so you can concentrate only on your form. If you are tall (over 5'10") and have a long torso, a good squat form is very difficult to master. Wear two belts to support your upper torso and protect against injury. Over the course of three months, you should work to be able to squat at 65% for 10-12 reps three times, then, work at 75% of your max for as many reps as possible once during the month, and finally, two other times, squat while holding whatever weight will allow you to complete 25 repetitions.

It is difficult to explain squatting techniques on paper, so you will be well advised to watch someone who is experienced performing the maneuver, or ask a trainer to help you. Keep in mind, you should never drop all the way down and then allow yourself to "bounce back," powered by the momentum created by you and the weight, Doing so can ruin your patella tendon (which connects the kneecap to the shin bone). Arch your lower back and keep your upper body as close to upright as possible. Never place the bar on your neck, rather rest it a little lower, on your traps, about 2-3 inches bellow the end of where the C-spine ends and where the T-spine begins. Keep your head up and watch your form in the mirror, if one is available. Monitor your movement; it should be fluid but rigid. Work to achieve one continuous motion, so that you are moving the weight up and down, like a piston. Do not lock your knees at the top of the squat, and work to maintain a constant rhythm of just breaking parallel and then moving back up just before the point where your knees could lock. Beginner and intermediate squatters can really benefit from a spotter during their form-perfecting days. Have the spotter always grab you from the front, just bellow your chest and pull you up and slightly back, slowly keeping pace with your motion.

2.) If you feel you are a great squatter try this. Be sure to a have spotter, do a warm-up set, and then do one more light set of 15 reps. Next, use a weight that will allow you to complete 12-15 reps, but instead of stopping at 12-15, push yourself to your muscle failure point. Try this twice a month, each time trying to complete one more rep. When you can complete new repetition ranges, add 10-15 pounds and begin the cycle again. The combination of a high number of reps and heavy weight will do wonders for your thighs. Aim to complete 25-50 non-stop reps.

The leg press is a great machine for increasing both one's weight and anaerobic capacity, because it allows the user to make fine adjustments to find just the right stroke and length for his or her particular body. If you are a beginner you work to identify the place where you get the most stimulation under the heaviest load, without using either too short a stroke or maxing-out. Build up both your weight and stroke length over time to increase both the duration and intensity of your sets.

Intermediate and advanced lifters can really make an impact in leg growth with leg presses, because the machine gives the user a great deal of control.

Your first concern should be to find the right range for your body on the machine. You should be positioned with your feet almost together, and expect your knees to touch your chest. Your seat location should be your next concern. To determine proper seat positioning, set the weight to your heaviest amount to date, and adjust the seat so that you can complete 10 full-range reps. Next, adjust the seat so that you can complete 15 reps without stopping. Work to be able to complete 20-25 reps without stopping before you add more weight. Maintain this pattern of adding reps and weights unless you have the seat adjusted all the way to the top where you are only moving a few inches during each rep. Though very small movements work well for the forearms, larger leg muscles do not benefit from such short movements. This process done properly, will help build your anaerobic capacity, something that very few natural body builders have mastered. Once your capacity has increased, you will notice much more leg development than you would have ever thought possible. After you've been working in this way for a while, try dropping the seat to its original notch to see what you can do. You will be amazed! You will find that you are now able to surpass your original weight by a great deal, in spite of the range of motion actually being longer. Do this once a month. Remember though, your goal is not to be concerned with where the seat is, or how much weight is being used, the goal is to find the "sweet spot" that maximizes every fiber in your thighs and it stimulates them to grow like never before. MMS is your ultimate goal!

Contrary to the thinking of the old paradigm, leg extensions are a good way to build your legs' frontal size. Don't think of them merely as a finishing exercise. Feel free to do leg extensions first, not just to warm up, but to place a good heavy load on your quadriceps before going on to the leg press and/or the squat rack. Leg extensions can do wonders for developing your quadriceps. As a rule of thumb, warm up lightly and then go right into a heavy set of 20 extensions, resting only a minute or so before starting another set with the same amount of weight. Do this three times. Don't ever drop the weight, but do consider finishing the last set with only about eight reps if that is where the cycle leads you. This is not to say that leg extensions cannot also be a good finishing exercise after doing squats and/or leg presses.

Leg extensions lend themselves well to people with long legs, and are helpful in combination with other multi-joint exercises in terms of strength-building, as the extensions help to increase blood flow to the legs before going onto squats and/or presses.

To get a really good leg workout, rely on one or two of these exercises: the squat, the leg press, the horizontal leg press, the hack squat, or leg extensions. Don't be afraid to change the order in which you perform the exercises – mix it up a bit! The hack squat and the horizontal leg press machines are also good for overall leg size. Be sure to use the same techniques in these exercises to find your proper range, rhythm, amount of weight, and number of sets, then substitute one of these for one of the three exercises outlined above. Above all, be sure that you don't overexert yourself with too many exercises, or else you will never be able to recover in time for your next leg workout, ideally held five to 15 days after your first leg day. Any sooner is too soon; anything after will see you run the risk of losing hypertrophy. You can see a dramatic improvement in your legs in a very short amount of time if you have the form and intensity down to a science. The key is to reach MMS with the fewest sets. This will come over a long period of trial and error, and great persistence and general awareness.

Leg Biceps

Although leg biceps usually grow as a result of proper squatting and high intensity leg pressing, it is a good idea to add leg curls with both legs, and/or one leg at a time to your routine. The key with these exercises is to pull with the leg biceps and not allow the gluteus maximus to engage during the performance of the set. When doing one-legged leg curls, be sure you tilt your upper body forward a bit, so as to apply maximum intensity on the leg biceps. In your mind's eye, think of the leg biceps as you think of your arm biceps – isolated during the set.

Another exercise that some may find helpful is the "stiff-legged dead lift." This can cause lower back problems and unless you are already familiar with it, and are capable of executing it properly (keeping your back flat and pulling up with stiff arms), then I would not recommend that you add this exercise to your routine.

Thinking about leg presses and squats in general, you will find that building strength and anaerobic endurance will give you far greater development for the leg biceps than relatively light, and oftentimes poorly executed, leg biceps curls.

Calves

Many people have difficulty developing their calves. In the old days, it was thought that calves should be worked every day; this was based on the idea that, since we are on our feet all the time, calves need a lot of extra stimulation in order to "grow" the way a bodybuilder would like.

Now we know that calves actually only need to be worked perhaps once per week. Sometimes rest is more important than a rigid workout routine. We know that muscles can change (from red to white or vice versa, all brought about by different training methods) over time, therefore, you should stretch a lot and participate in a martial art, play a recreational sport, or some other type of non-weight-oriented exercise, so that the muscles do not become rigid, capable only of lifting weights.

Bodybuilders who stopped the constant calf training regimen in favor of weekly training sessions have reported sudden bursts of growth, not only because they broke the cycle of over-training, but also because they implemented a more biomechanically correct training program. A near-instant, positive response was their reward.

Whenever you refer back to an old Schwarzenegger routine or another of the Weider promotional workout directives, you will find advice concerning the importance of training calves everyday and other nuggets of information that have since been proven less than ideal for natural weightlifting practitioners. You must remember, most of the athletes profiled in the Weider publications of old were on steroids. The muscle recovery time for those taking steroids is at least twice as fast as those not on anabolics, all because of the increase in protein synthesis, carbohydrate uptake, Krebs cycle modifications and faster soft tissue repair, all hallmarks of the steroid effects on the body.

Ironically, oftentimes training calves 3x per week for three months rather than training them the once per week, works for some "natural" men over 40. It is a shame to note that this seemingly instant muscle growth that follows periods of decreased calf training only holds true for the calves themselves. I have experimented with this notion in other muscle groups, but only observed atrophy and no positive rebounding effects after the everyday routines were halted. Training calves can be tricky. Some people will achieve great calves very easily, thanks to great genetics, but anyone who is willing to work very hard to improve weak calves can bring them up. I recommend that you train your calves very intensely every time you work your legs. When performing standing calf raises, or any other calf exercise, really squeeze your calves and hold them firm at the top of the repetition. As with all muscle groups, try several variations of exercises and intense sets, sometimes only moving the calves up and down no more than an inch, for as long as you can stand it. Do this only after a full regular set of calf work. If you are interested in predicting your potential calf size and shape, you need look no further than where your calves attach to your lower legs and ankles: these are your bio-mechanical predictors. The lower the attachment point, the bigger and fuller your calves are inherently; the larger your knees, and especially your ankles, the greater your potential for good-sized calves. Also, the thickness and width of your achilles tendon can be of some help in seeing the potentiality for the calves. Like other muscles, the shape of your calves is largely determined within your DNA shape and and joint sizes. Do not let these indicators deter you; even those who have high attachments can develop great calves. Yours may require more experimentation than average, but that is all. Where there is a will there is way, no matter what your genetic predisposition.

Bringing It All Together

With the completion of this chapter, you should have a good feeling of familiarity with the subtleties of weight training, your own body and which exercises you should do for each of your unique body parts. And, equally as important, you should know when to rest, when to go all out after MMS and when to walk or swim, or simply relax.

Hopefully you have also begun to uncover the answers to questions you have had about weight training but have never before been able to deduce them yourself.

Now Let's Take a Look at All These Exercises Through Illustrations.....

(Although not all exercise illustrations show exerciser with a belt; it is imperative to wear a weight training belt while doing all weight training movements. The only time you don't wear a belt is while doing waist or hyperextensions.)

Upright Rows

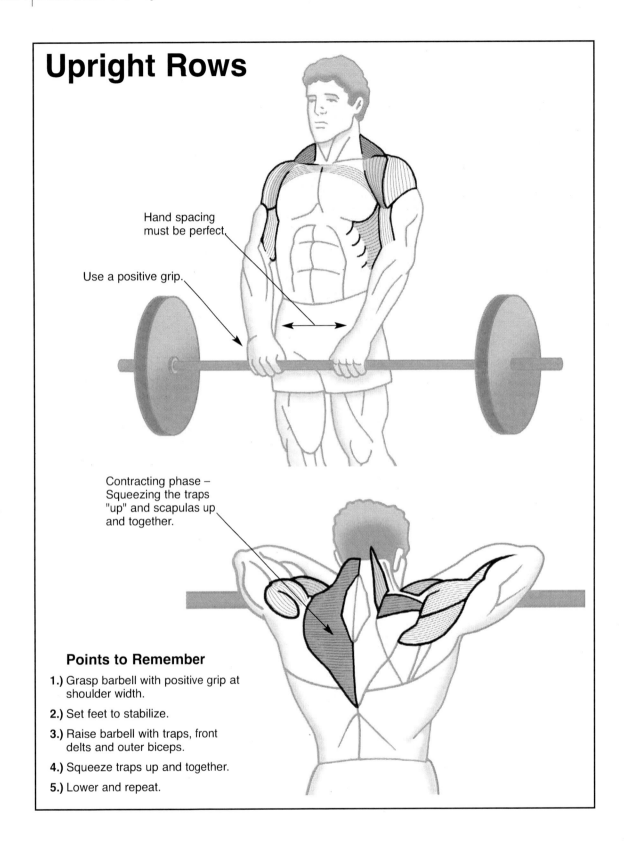

Hand spacing must be perfect.

Use a positive grip.

Contracting phase – Squeezing the traps "up" and scapulas up and together.

Points to Remember

1.) Grasp barbell with positive grip at shoulder width.

2.) Set feet to stabilize.

3.) Raise barbell with traps, front delts and outer biceps.

4.) Squeeze traps up and together.

5.) Lower and repeat.

Bent Over Rows

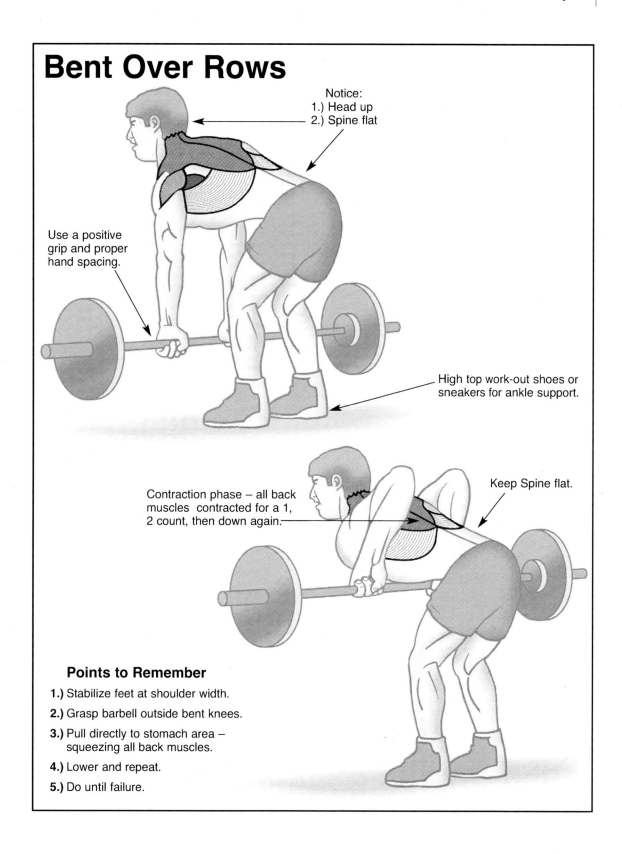

Notice:
1.) Head up
2.) Spine flat

Use a positive grip and proper hand spacing.

High top work-out shoes or sneakers for ankle support.

Contraction phase – all back muscles contracted for a 1, 2 count, then down again.

Keep Spine flat.

Points to Remember

1.) Stabilize feet at shoulder width.

2.) Grasp barbell outside bent knees.

3.) Pull directly to stomach area – squeezing all back muscles.

4.) Lower and repeat.

5.) Do until failure.

Barbell Shoulder Shrugs

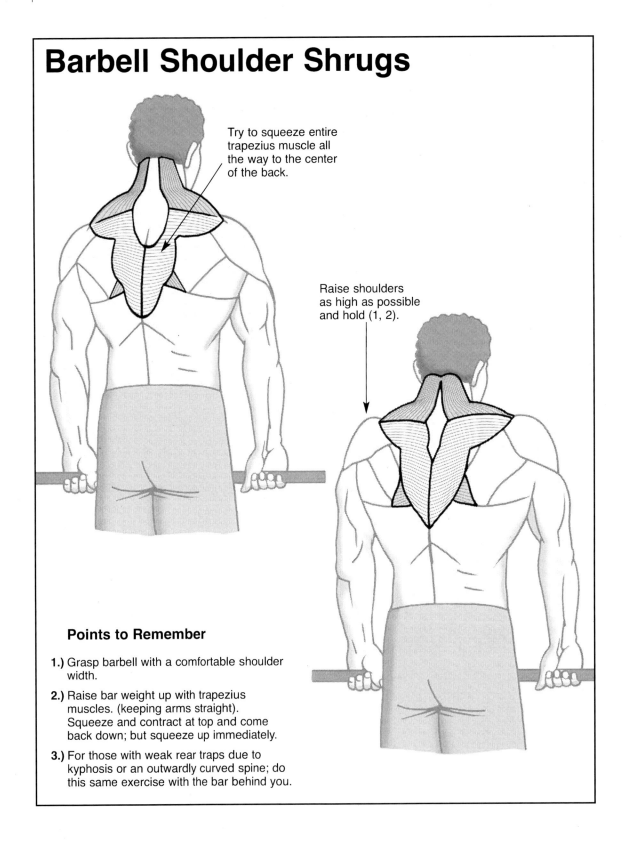

Try to squeeze entire trapezius muscle all the way to the center of the back.

Raise shoulders as high as possible and hold (1, 2).

Points to Remember

1.) Grasp barbell with a comfortable shoulder width.

2.) Raise bar weight up with trapezius muscles. (keeping arms straight). Squeeze and contract at top and come back down; but squeeze up immediately.

3.) For those with weak rear traps due to kyphosis or an outwardly curved spine; do this same exercise with the bar behind you.

Seated Dumbbell Presses

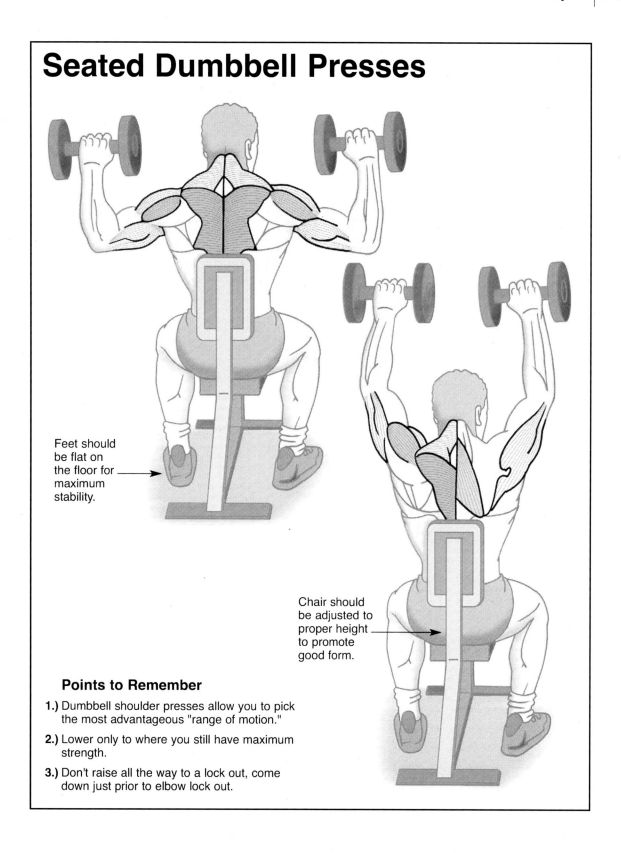

Feet should be flat on the floor for maximum stability.

Chair should be adjusted to proper height to promote good form.

Points to Remember

1.) Dumbbell shoulder presses allow you to pick the most advantageous "range of motion."

2.) Lower only to where you still have maximum strength.

3.) Don't raise all the way to a lock out, come down just prior to elbow lock out.

Bent Over Lateral Raises

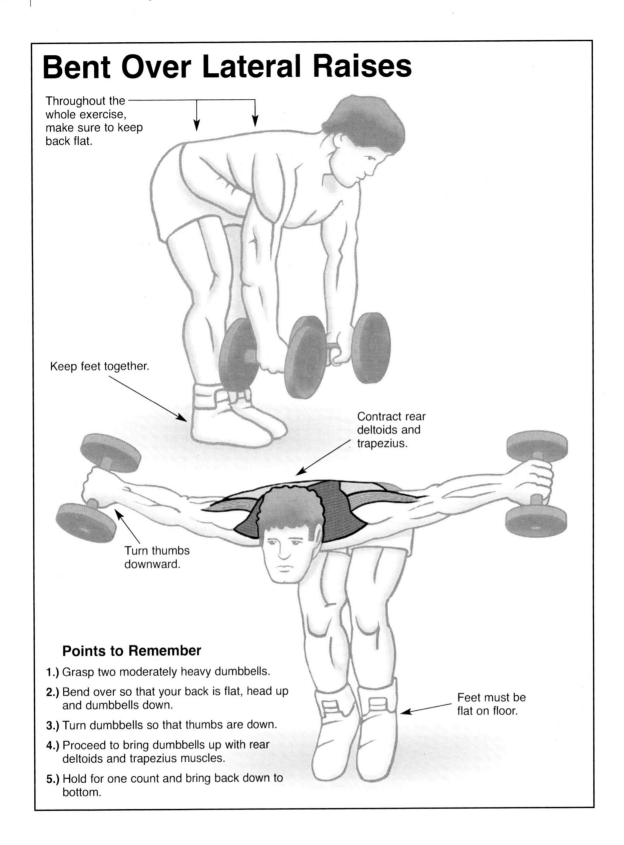

Throughout the whole exercise, make sure to keep back flat.

Keep feet together.

Contract rear deltoids and trapezius.

Turn thumbs downward.

Feet must be flat on floor.

Points to Remember

1.) Grasp two moderately heavy dumbbells.

2.) Bend over so that your back is flat, head up and dumbbells down.

3.) Turn dumbbells so that thumbs are down.

4.) Proceed to bring dumbbells up with rear deltoids and trapezius muscles.

5.) Hold for one count and bring back down to bottom.

Front Pull Downs

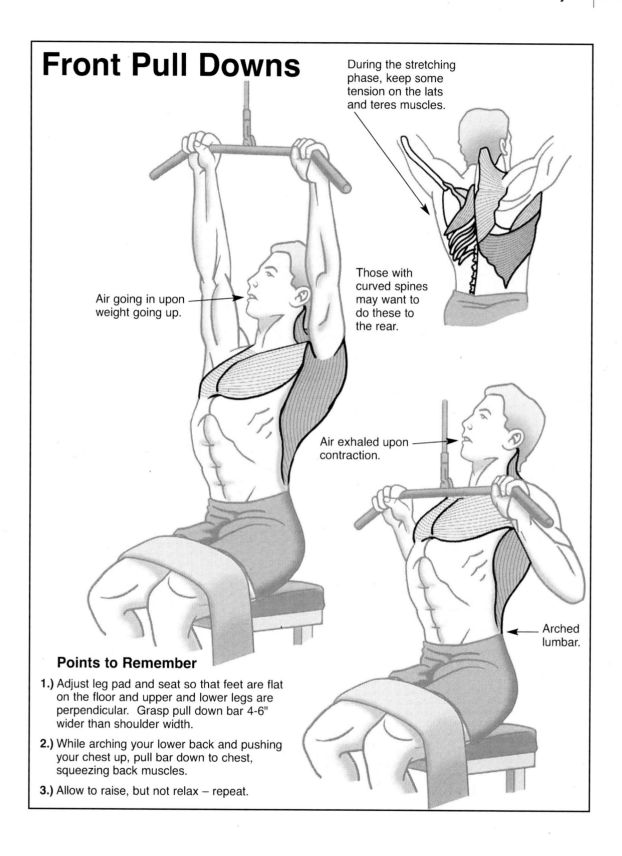

During the stretching phase, keep some tension on the lats and teres muscles.

Those with curved spines may want to do these to the rear.

Air going in upon weight going up.

Air exhaled upon contraction.

Arched lumbar.

Points to Remember

1.) Adjust leg pad and seat so that feet are flat on the floor and upper and lower legs are perpendicular. Grasp pull down bar 4-6" wider than shoulder width.

2.) While arching your lower back and pushing your chest up, pull bar down to chest, squeezing back muscles.

3.) Allow to raise, but not relax – repeat.

Pull Ups

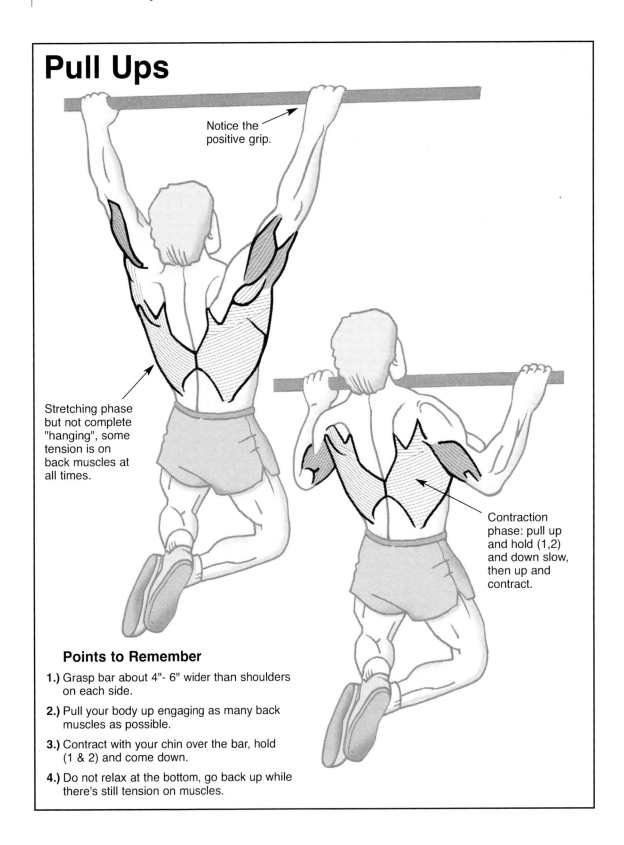

Notice the positive grip.

Stretching phase but not complete "hanging", some tension is on back muscles at all times.

Contraction phase: pull up and hold (1,2) and down slow, then up and contract.

Points to Remember

1.) Grasp bar about 4"- 6" wider than shoulders on each side.

2.) Pull your body up engaging as many back muscles as possible.

3.) Contract with your chin over the bar, hold (1 & 2) and come down.

4.) Do not relax at the bottom, go back up while there's still tension on muscles.

Cable Cross Overs

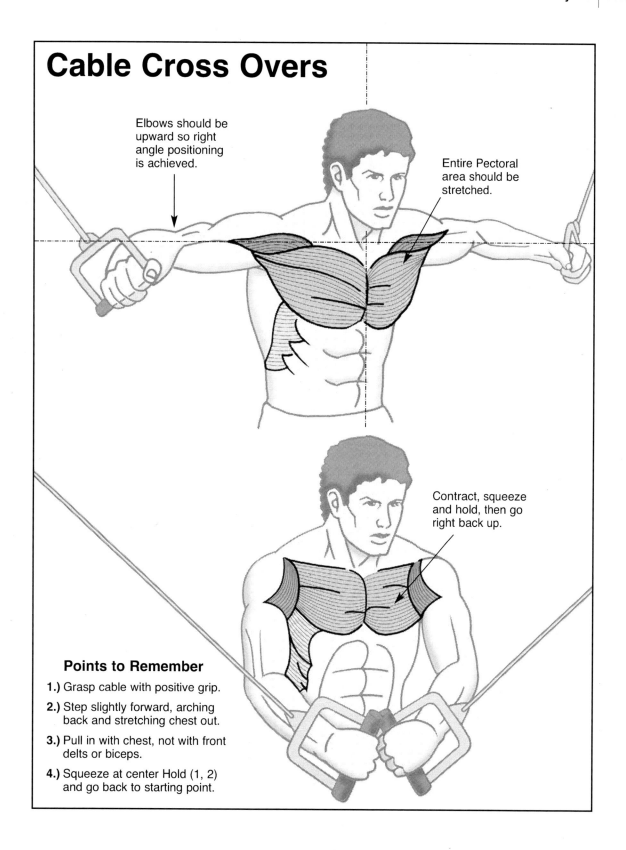

Elbows should be upward so right angle positioning is achieved.

Entire Pectoral area should be stretched.

Contract, squeeze and hold, then go right back up.

Points to Remember

1.) Grasp cable with positive grip.

2.) Step slightly forward, arching back and stretching chest out.

3.) Pull in with chest, not with front delts or biceps.

4.) Squeeze at center Hold (1, 2) and go back to starting point.

Reverse Grip Pull Downs

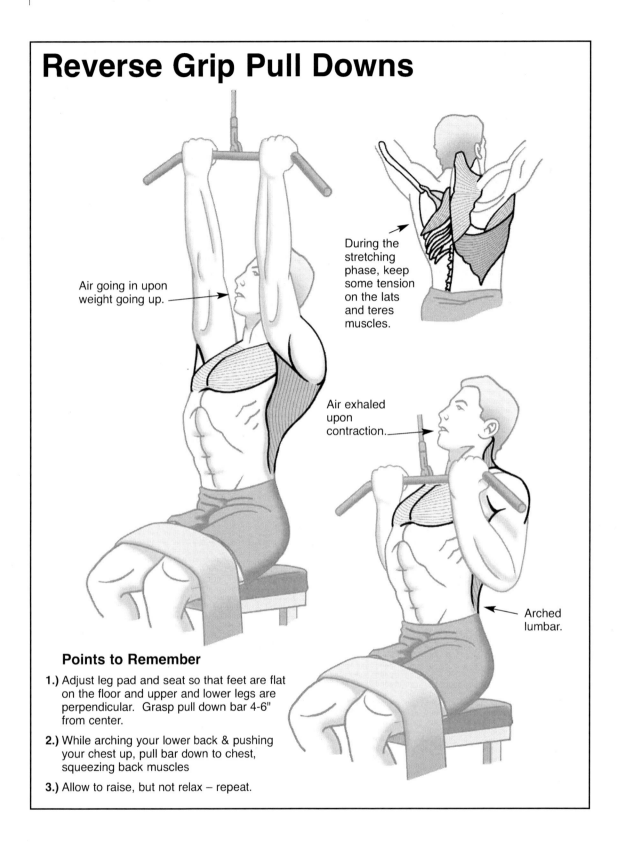

Air going in upon weight going up.

During the stretching phase, keep some tension on the lats and teres muscles.

Air exhaled upon contraction.

Arched lumbar.

Points to Remember

1.) Adjust leg pad and seat so that feet are flat on the floor and upper and lower legs are perpendicular. Grasp pull down bar 4-6" from center.

2.) While arching your lower back & pushing your chest up, pull bar down to chest, squeezing back muscles

3.) Allow to raise, but not relax – repeat.

Front Dumbbell Raises

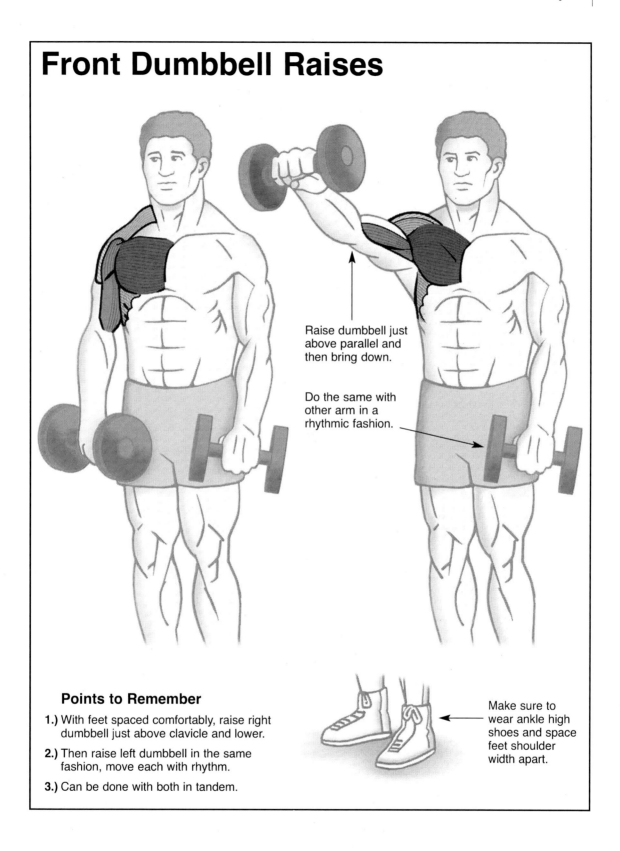

Raise dumbbell just above parallel and then bring down.

Do the same with other arm in a rhythmic fashion.

Points to Remember

1.) With feet spaced comfortably, raise right dumbbell just above clavicle and lower.

2.) Then raise left dumbbell in the same fashion, move each with rhythm.

3.) Can be done with both in tandem.

Make sure to wear ankle high shoes and space feet shoulder width apart.

Flat Bench Dumbbell Presses

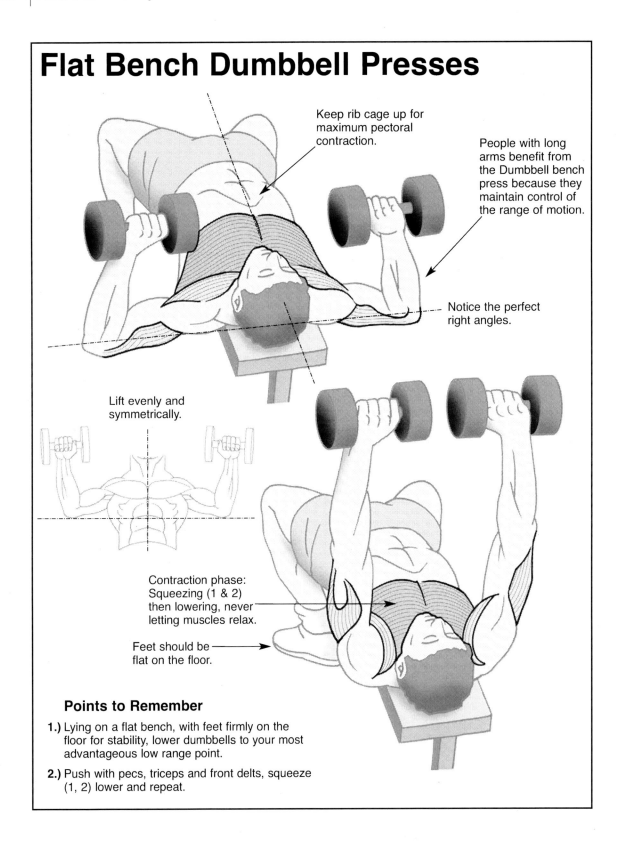

Keep rib cage up for maximum pectoral contraction.

People with long arms benefit from the Dumbbell bench press because they maintain control of the range of motion.

Notice the perfect right angles.

Lift evenly and symmetrically.

Contraction phase: Squeezing (1 & 2) then lowering, never letting muscles relax.

Feet should be flat on the floor.

Points to Remember

1.) Lying on a flat bench, with feet firmly on the floor for stability, lower dumbbells to your most advantageous low range point.

2.) Push with pecs, triceps and front delts, squeeze (1, 2) lower and repeat.

Decline Dumbbell Presses

Excellent exercise for those with long arms and/or who have difficulties bench pressing with bar.

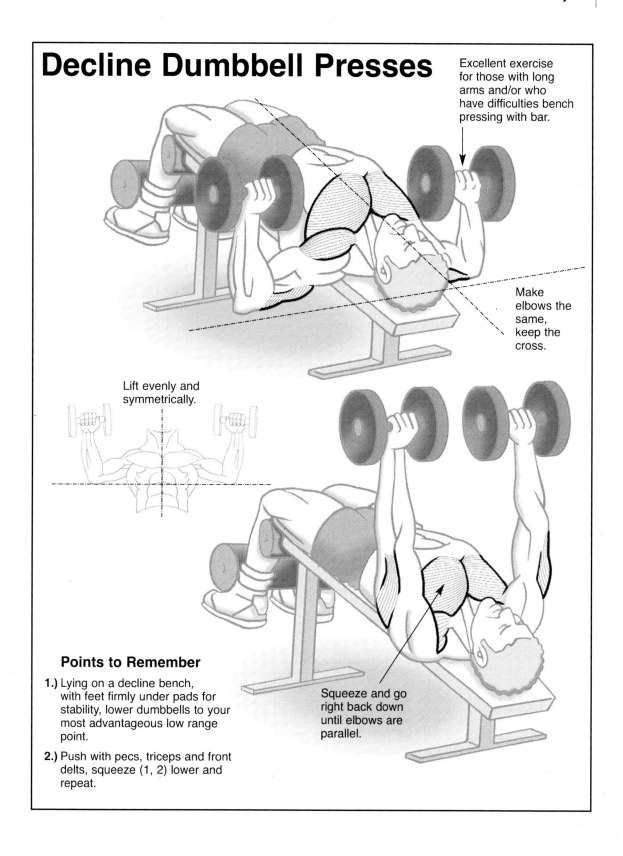

Make elbows the same, keep the cross.

Lift evenly and symmetrically.

Squeeze and go right back down until elbows are parallel.

Points to Remember

1.) Lying on a decline bench, with feet firmly under pads for stability, lower dumbbells to your most advantageous low range point.

2.) Push with pecs, triceps and front delts, squeeze (1, 2) lower and repeat.

Flat Bench Dumbbell Flye

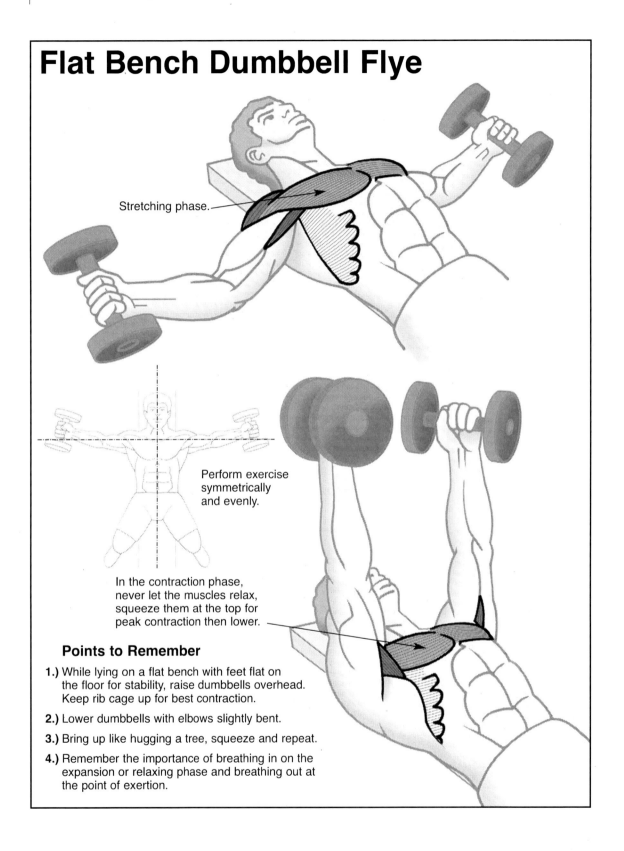

Stretching phase.

Perform exercise symmetrically and evenly.

In the contraction phase, never let the muscles relax, squeeze them at the top for peak contraction then lower.

Points to Remember

1.) While lying on a flat bench with feet flat on the floor for stability, raise dumbbells overhead. Keep rib cage up for best contraction.

2.) Lower dumbbells with elbows slightly bent.

3.) Bring up like hugging a tree, squeeze and repeat.

4.) Remember the importance of breathing in on the expansion or relaxing phase and breathing out at the point of exertion.

Seated Chest Machine Presses

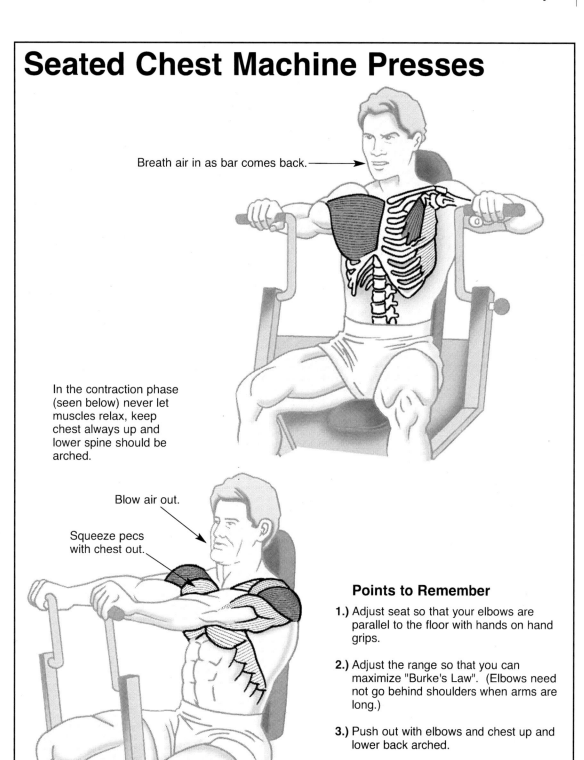

Breath air in as bar comes back.

In the contraction phase (seen below) never let muscles relax, keep chest always up and lower spine should be arched.

Blow air out.

Squeeze pecs with chest out.

Points to Remember

1.) Adjust seat so that your elbows are parallel to the floor with hands on hand grips.

2.) Adjust the range so that you can maximize "Burke's Law". (Elbows need not go behind shoulders when arms are long.)

3.) Push out with elbows and chest up and lower back arched.

4.) Squeeze pecs for one count and return to point of maximum leverage.

Inclined Dumbbell Presses

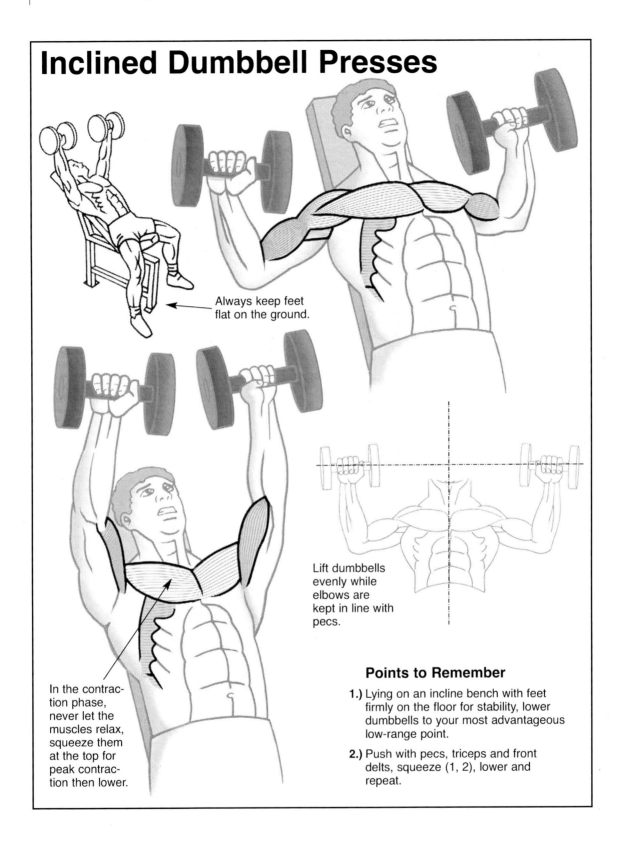

Always keep feet flat on the ground.

Lift dumbbells evenly while elbows are kept in line with pecs.

In the contraction phase, never let the muscles relax, squeeze them at the top for peak contraction then lower.

Points to Remember

1.) Lying on an incline bench with feet firmly on the floor for stability, lower dumbbells to your most advantageous low-range point.

2.) Push with pecs, triceps and front delts, squeeze (1, 2), lower and repeat.

114

Seated Cable Rows

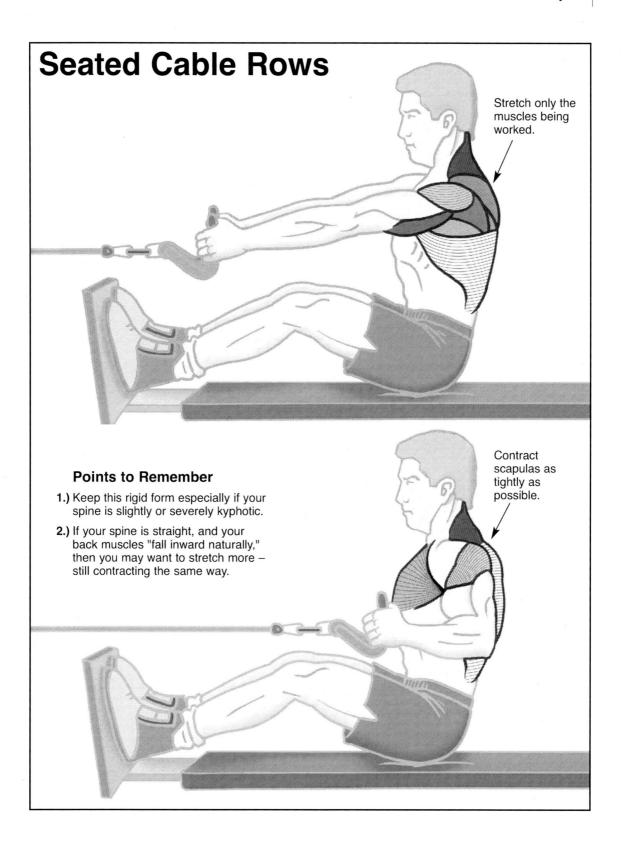

Stretch only the muscles being worked.

Contract scapulas as tightly as possible.

Points to Remember

1.) Keep this rigid form especially if your spine is slightly or severely kyphotic.

2.) If your spine is straight, and your back muscles "fall inward naturally," then you may want to stretch more – still contracting the same way.

45° French Presses

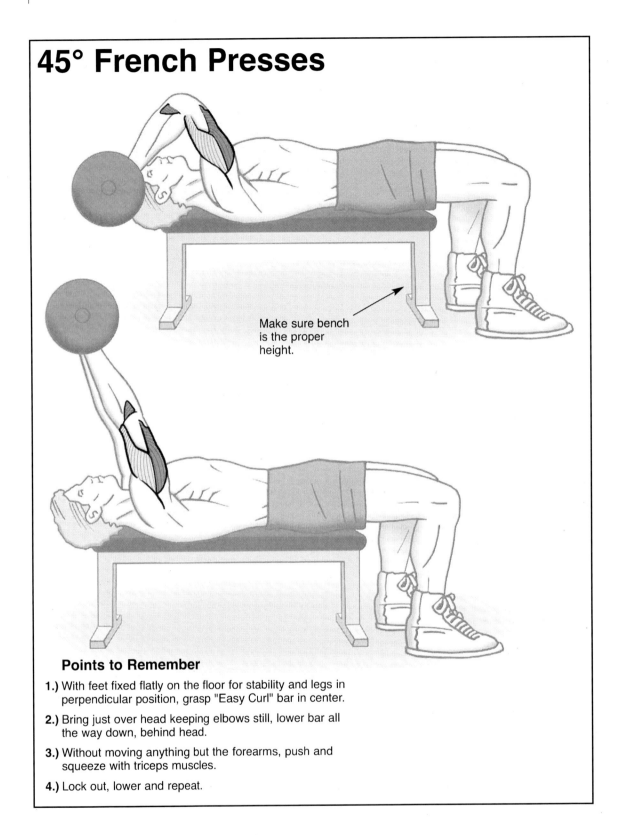

Make sure bench is the proper height.

Points to Remember

1.) With feet fixed flatly on the floor for stability and legs in perpendicular position, grasp "Easy Curl" bar in center.

2.) Bring just over head keeping elbows still, lower bar all the way down, behind head.

3.) Without moving anything but the forearms, push and squeeze with triceps muscles.

4.) Lock out, lower and repeat.

Overhead Tricep Presses

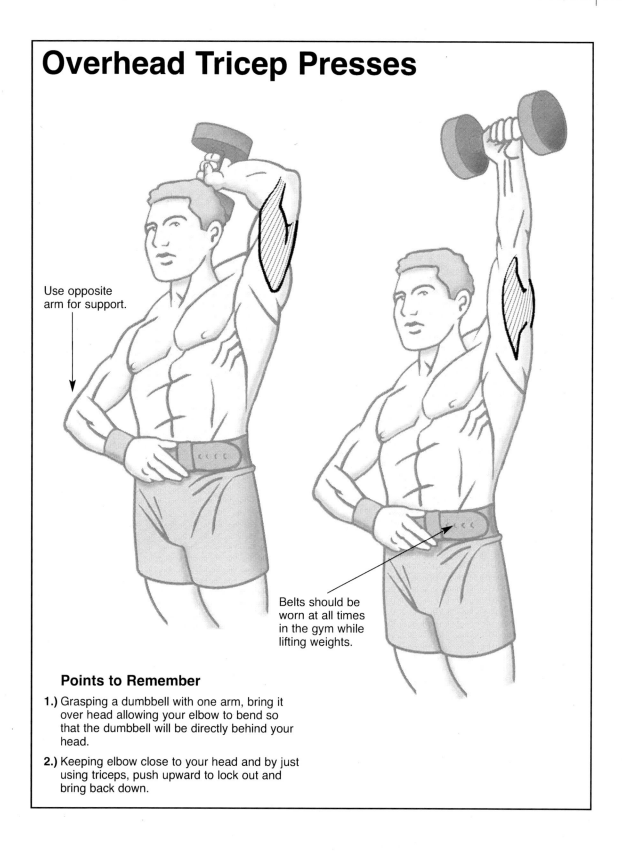

Use opposite arm for support.

Belts should be worn at all times in the gym while lifting weights.

Points to Remember

1.) Grasping a dumbbell with one arm, bring it over head allowing your elbow to bend so that the dumbbell will be directly behind your head.

2.) Keeping elbow close to your head and by just using triceps, push upward to lock out and bring back down.

Bar & Cable Push Downs

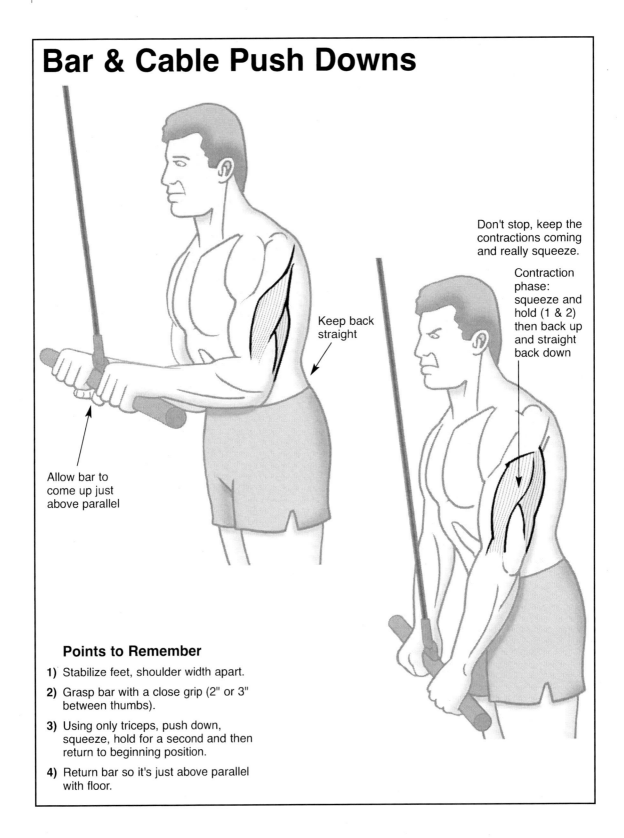

Keep back straight

Allow bar to come up just above parallel

Don't stop, keep the contractions coming and really squeeze.

Contraction phase: squeeze and hold (1 & 2) then back up and straight back down

Points to Remember

1) Stabilize feet, shoulder width apart.

2) Grasp bar with a close grip (2" or 3" between thumbs).

3) Using only triceps, push down, squeeze, hold for a second and then return to beginning position.

4) Return bar so it's just above parallel with floor.

Concentration Curls on Bench

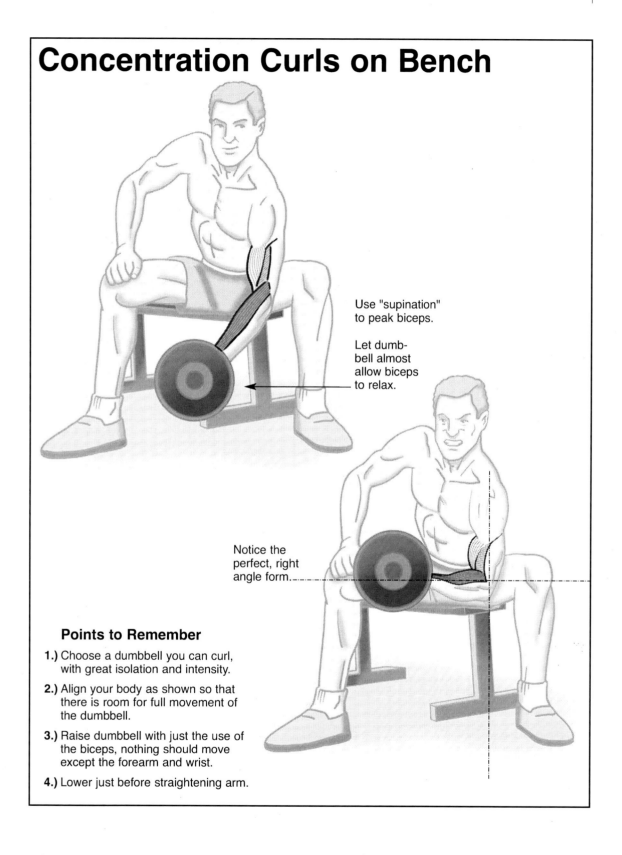

Use "supination" to peak biceps.

Let dumb-bell almost allow biceps to relax.

Notice the perfect, right angle form.

Points to Remember

1.) Choose a dumbbell you can curl, with great isolation and intensity.

2.) Align your body as shown so that there is room for full movement of the dumbbell.

3.) Raise dumbbell with just the use of the biceps, nothing should move except the forearm and wrist.

4.) Lower just before straightening arm.

Preacher Curls

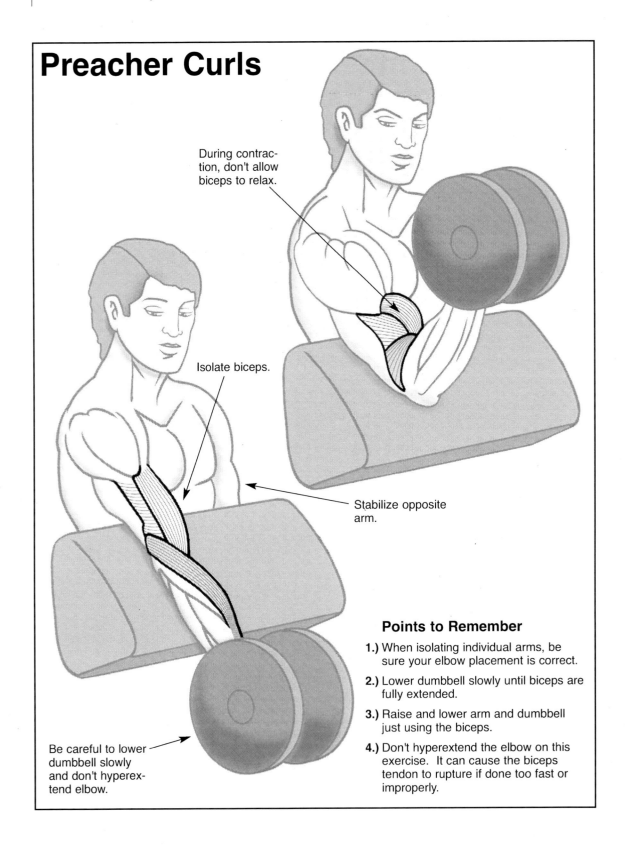

During contraction, don't allow biceps to relax.

Isolate biceps.

Stabilize opposite arm.

Be careful to lower dumbbell slowly and don't hyperextend elbow.

Points to Remember

1.) When isolating individual arms, be sure your elbow placement is correct.

2.) Lower dumbbell slowly until biceps are fully extended.

3.) Raise and lower arm and dumbbell just using the biceps.

4.) Don't hyperextend the elbow on this exercise. It can cause the biceps tendon to rupture if done too fast or improperly.

Standing Barbell Curls

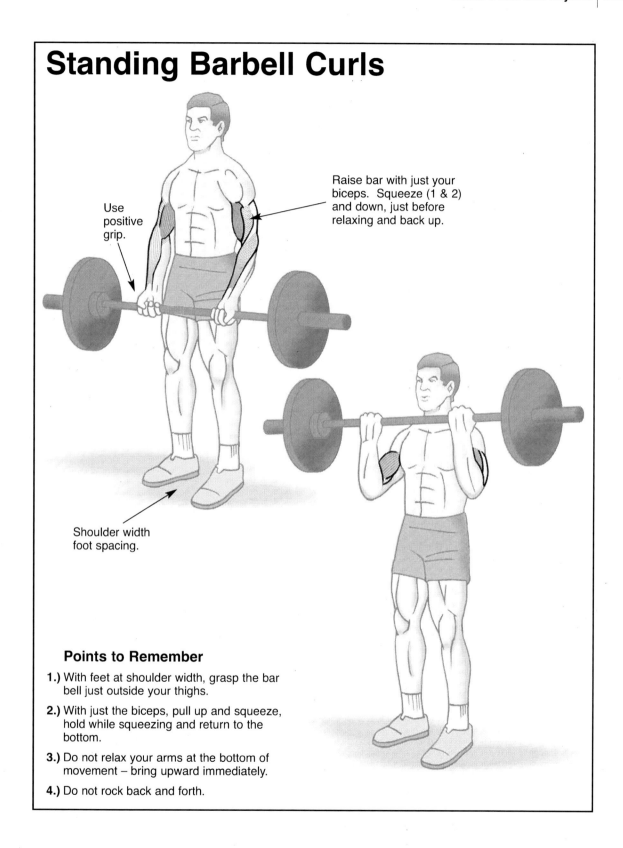

Use positive grip.

Raise bar with just your biceps. Squeeze (1 & 2) and down, just before relaxing and back up.

Shoulder width foot spacing.

Points to Remember

1.) With feet at shoulder width, grasp the bar bell just outside your thighs.

2.) With just the biceps, pull up and squeeze, hold while squeezing and return to the bottom.

3.) Do not relax your arms at the bottom of movement – bring upward immediately.

4.) Do not rock back and forth.

Dumbbell Wrist Curls

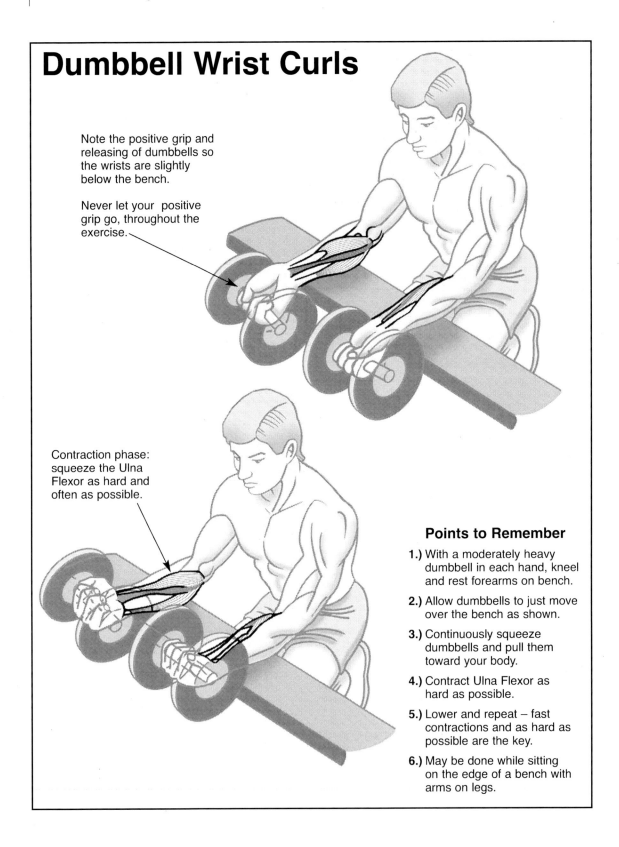

Note the positive grip and releasing of dumbbells so the wrists are slightly below the bench.

Never let your positive grip go, throughout the exercise.

Contraction phase: squeeze the Ulna Flexor as hard and often as possible.

Points to Remember

1.) With a moderately heavy dumbbell in each hand, kneel and rest forearms on bench.

2.) Allow dumbbells to just move over the bench as shown.

3.) Continuously squeeze dumbbells and pull them toward your body.

4.) Contract Ulna Flexor as hard as possible.

5.) Lower and repeat – fast contractions and as hard as possible are the key.

6.) May be done while sitting on the edge of a bench with arms on legs.

Reverse Abdominal Crunches

Air in.

Air out upon contraction.

Squeeze both upper and lower abdominals.

Points to Remember

1.) Lying on a flat, or inclined bench.

2.) Keep back as straight as possible pull straight up to just before the knees hit the chest.

3.) Drop down and repeat.

4.) Use both the upper and lower abdominal regions.

Hanging Knee Raises

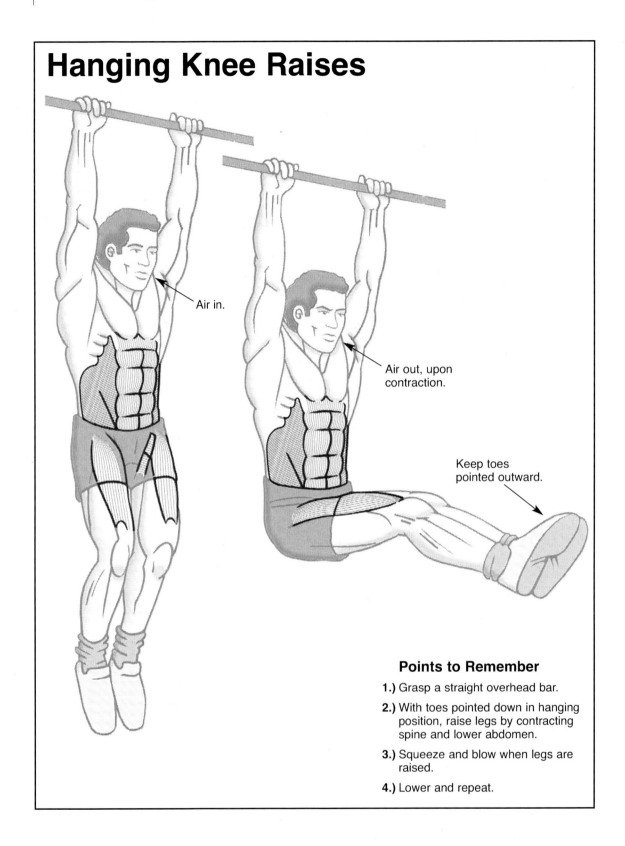

Air in.

Air out, upon contraction.

Keep toes pointed outward.

Points to Remember

1.) Grasp a straight overhead bar.

2.) With toes pointed down in hanging position, raise legs by contracting spine and lower abdomen.

3.) Squeeze and blow when legs are raised.

4.) Lower and repeat.

Barbell Squats

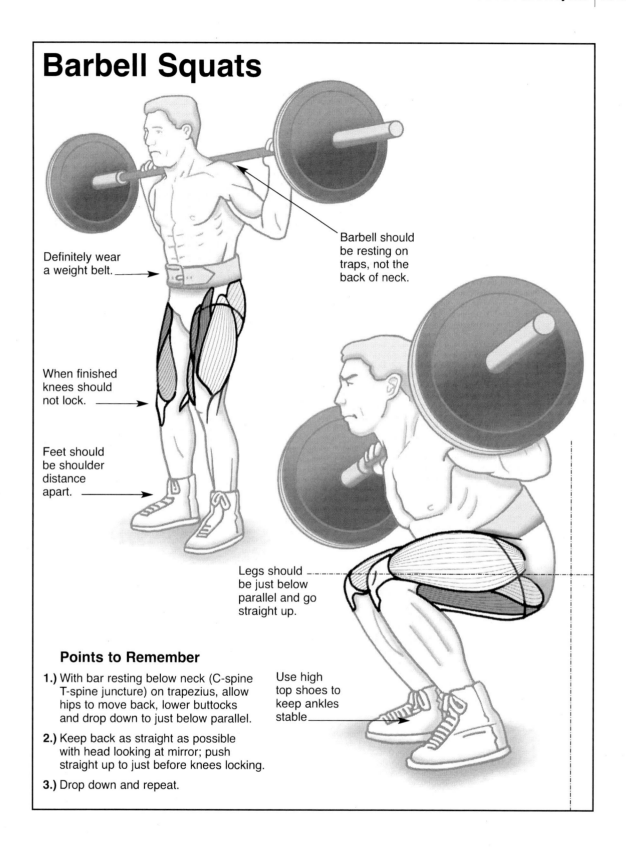

Definitely wear a weight belt.

Barbell should be resting on traps, not the back of neck.

When finished knees should not lock.

Feet should be shoulder distance apart.

Legs should be just below parallel and go straight up.

Points to Remember

1.) With bar resting below neck (C-spine T-spine juncture) on trapezius, allow hips to move back, lower buttocks and drop down to just below parallel.

2.) Keep back as straight as possible with head looking at mirror; push straight up to just before knees locking.

3.) Drop down and repeat.

Use high top shoes to keep ankles stable

Leg Extensions

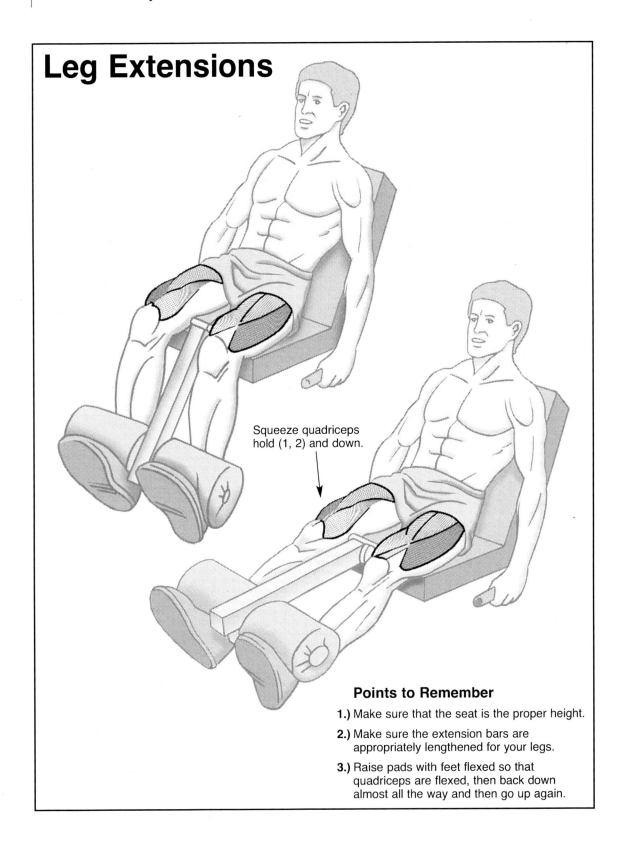

Squeeze quadriceps hold (1, 2) and down.

Points to Remember

1.) Make sure that the seat is the proper height.

2.) Make sure the extension bars are appropriately lengthened for your legs.

3.) Raise pads with feet flexed so that quadriceps are flexed, then back down almost all the way and then go up again.

Stiff Legged Dead Lifts

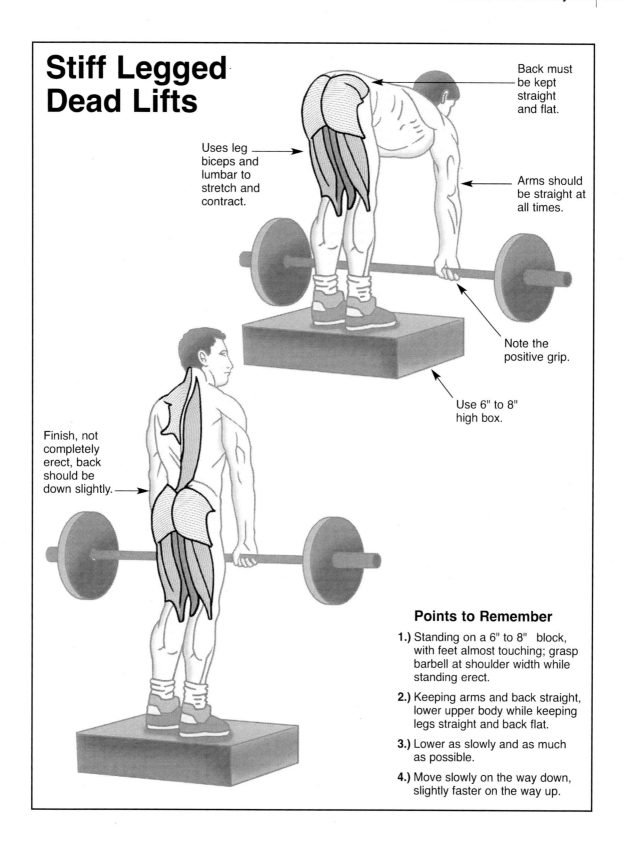

Back must be kept straight and flat.

Uses leg biceps and lumbar to stretch and contract.

Arms should be straight at all times.

Note the positive grip.

Use 6" to 8" high box.

Finish, not completely erect, back should be down slightly.

Points to Remember

1.) Standing on a 6" to 8" block, with feet almost touching; grasp barbell at shoulder width while standing erect.

2.) Keeping arms and back straight, lower upper body while keeping legs straight and back flat.

3.) Lower as slowly and as much as possible.

4.) Move slowly on the way down, slightly faster on the way up.

Lying Leg Curls

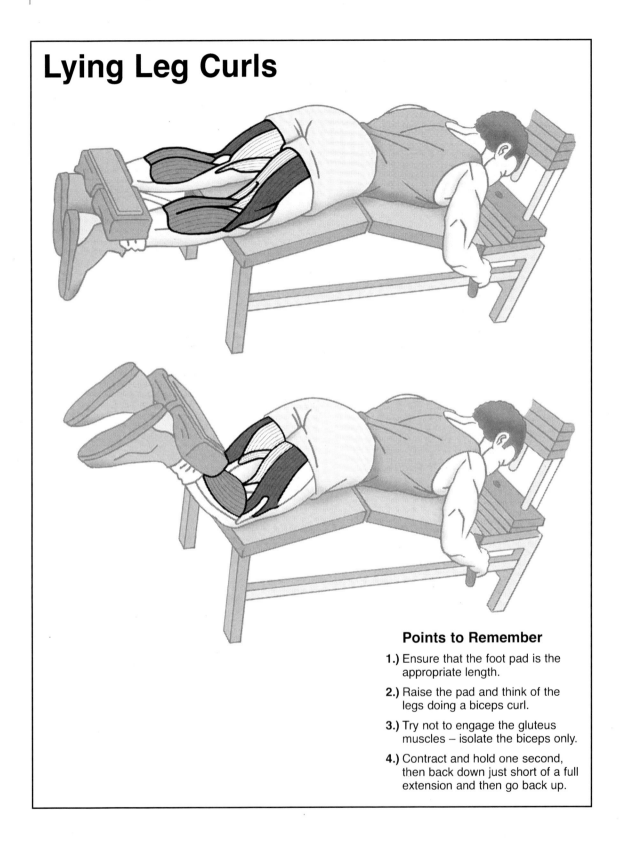

Points to Remember

1.) Ensure that the foot pad is the appropriate length.

2.) Raise the pad and think of the legs doing a biceps curl.

3.) Try not to engage the gluteus muscles – isolate the biceps only.

4.) Contract and hold one second, then back down just short of a full extension and then go back up.

Leg Presses

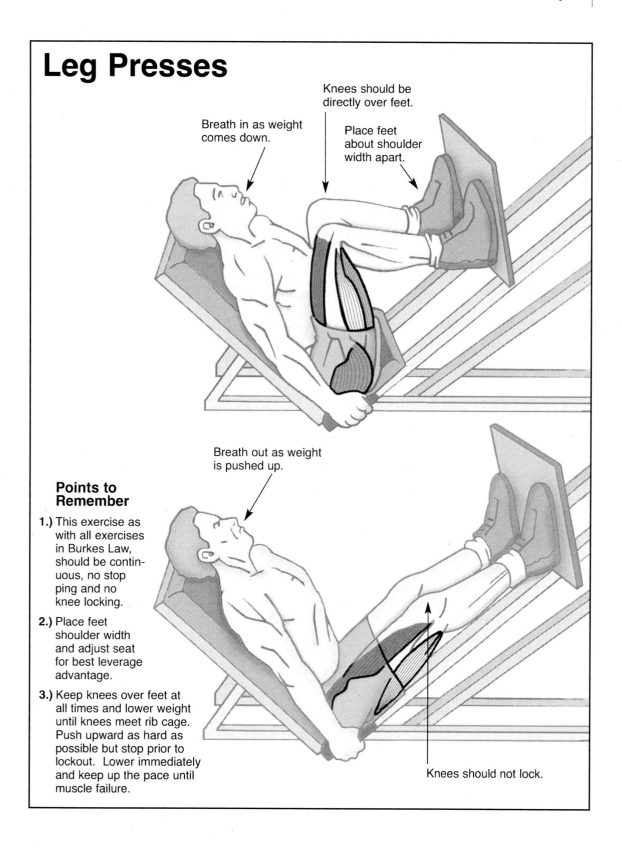

Knees should be directly over feet.

Breath in as weight comes down.

Place feet about shoulder width apart.

Breath out as weight is pushed up.

Knees should not lock.

Points to Remember

1.) This exercise as with all exercises in Burkes Law, should be continuous, no stopping and no knee locking.

2.) Place feet shoulder width and adjust seat for best leverage advantage.

3.) Keep knees over feet at all times and lower weight until knees meet rib cage. Push upward as hard as possible but stop prior to lockout. Lower immediately and keep up the pace until muscle failure.

Standing Calf Raises

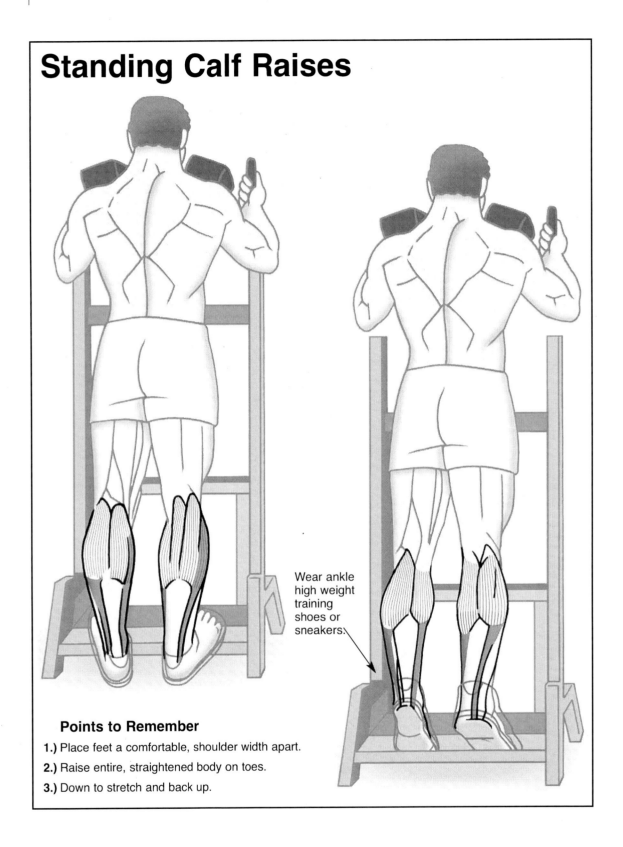

Wear ankle high weight training shoes or sneakers.

Points to Remember

1.) Place feet a comfortable, shoulder width apart.

2.) Raise entire, straightened body on toes.

3.) Down to stretch and back up.

Seated Calve Raises

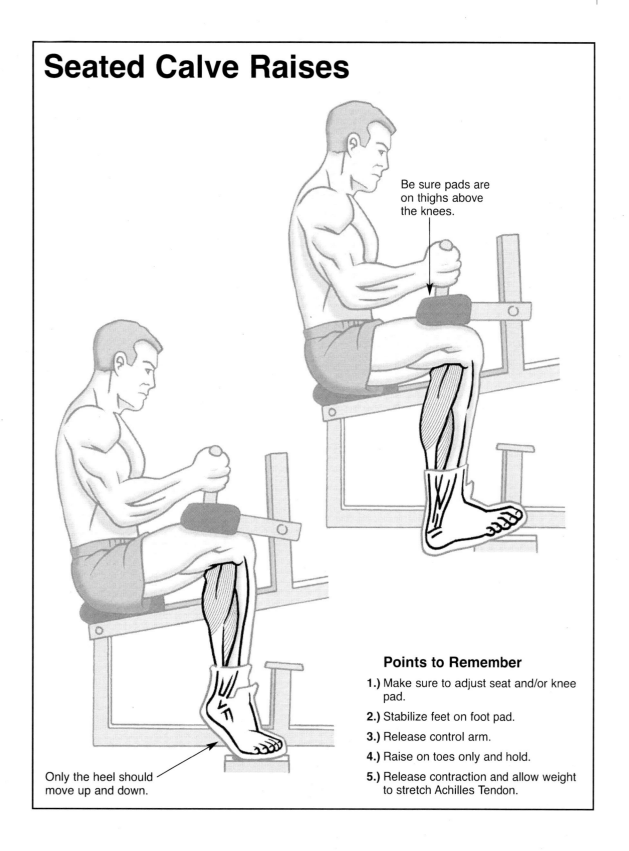

Be sure pads are on thighs above the knees.

Only the heel should move up and down.

Points to Remember

1.) Make sure to adjust seat and/or knee pad.

2.) Stabilize feet on foot pad.

3.) Release control arm.

4.) Raise on toes only and hold.

5.) Release contraction and allow weight to stretch Achilles Tendon.

Toe Raises

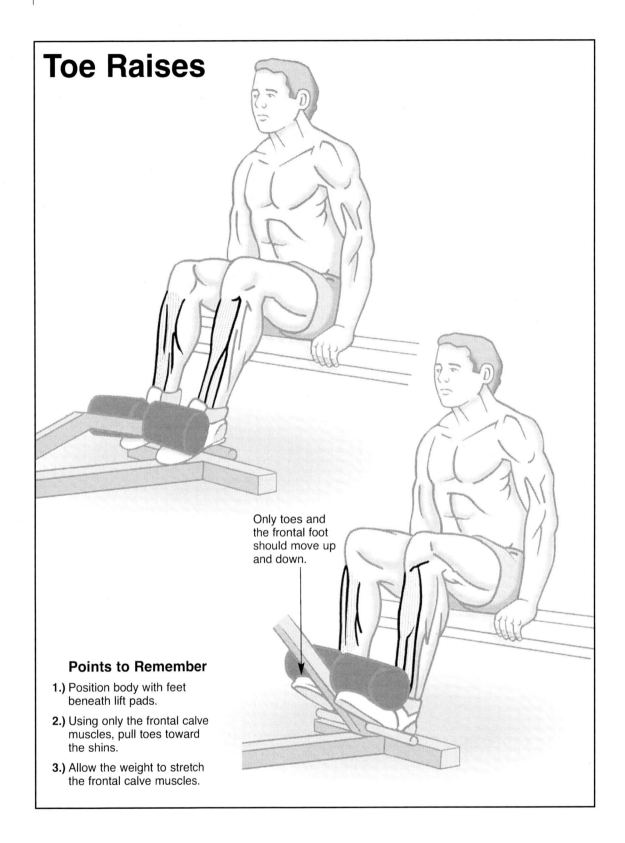

Only toes and
the frontal foot
should move up
and down.

Points to Remember

1.) Position body with feet
beneath lift pads.

2.) Using only the frontal calve
muscles, pull toes toward
the shins.

3.) Allow the weight to stretch
the frontal calve muscles.

Notes:

Notes:

5 | Injuries and What to do About Them When You Get Them

Injuries That Seem to Be Inevitable
with "Old Paradigm" Training

When most people begin lifting weights, they experience soreness and long delays between workouts – they take it slow and are careful with their body. I highly recommend this when beginning Burke's Law training; whether you are a novice or an advanced weight trainer or bodybuilder.

Unfortunately, most men I have noticed seem to forget the carefulness in which they began or begin new programs. They start to look at seasoned bodybuilders and mimic them. This ego chase, I have mentioned seems to go on in a lot of gyms. The major problem is that bodybuilding and fitness are not Power Lifting, nor Olympic Lifting. In other words, what one person with a certain frame can bench press (as demonstrated in Chapter 13) and another person with a less advantageous frame can bench press is not only going to be different; but it will never change (unless people resort to large amounts of growth hormone, or illegal anabolic steroids). In other words, injuries are usually from a poor choice in exercise for the body part and/or an ego-based training competition that secretly goes on between men in gyms.

The most common injury I have seen in bodybuilding is by far the various shoulder injuries that can occur. The barbell bench press for some is as easy as shuffling cards; but even for them if they become cocky and they use too much weight they will either hurt the tendons in the deltoid area; or temporarily (and/or permanently) injure the AC (acrominioclavicular) joint(s). Under each shoulder is a very complex group of ligaments, bursa sacks, cartilage and bones that connect and form the tremendously versatile human shoulder. The human body is a truly amazing evolution of joints and articulations that allow for throwing a baseball at the speed of one hundred miles an hour; or swim hundreds of meters in the "butterfly" stroke. The shoulder joints are incredibly versatile; however, they are not the same strength in each of us. The human shoulder allows us to do weight lifting exercises as extreme as flies and as simple as pressing; yet, nothing will rip that amazingly complex piece of evolution faster than constantly heavy bench pressing.

Bench pressing is good for some: Those with a leverage advantage and have no shoulder, elbow or wrist problems. On the other hand, many people should not bench press at all. Most people have a response to this such as "Arnold did them and his chest was huge." If you are still thinking this way, you have missed the point of the book. You must find the best exercises for each body part relative to your leverage advantage and ease of mastering proper form within each particular body part.

If you feel any "pinching" or "aching" in any joint, stop immediately. Then you should be able to diagnose the injury yourself based on your growing knowledge of your biomechanics and your form during exercise.

The most common problem with the shoulders (and many joint areas) is tendinitis. This is the inflammation of the inner mobile tissue of the tendon; and, the outer shell is shrinking at the same time. Rest is your first course of action. Then, when the pain begins to subside, begin to work the shoulder area with light dumbbells for high repetitions (30-40). Immediately after, you should learn and practice the daily shoulder tendon stretching exercise. This is executed by moving the right hand upside down as you move it out at shoulder level, then at arms length, reverse the move of the right hand and begin that movement with the left. It should become a fluid movement. After doing this for at least two minutes, put direct ice to the area for twenty minutes on and twenty off for three consecutive times. In a month, or less, your tendinitis will heal. Do not go back into doing heavy movements with the shoulder; instead, work your way back slowly and be aware that you are prone to this problem in this joint.

AC Inflammation: This is usually from bench pressing too heavy; cheating your hands out too wide on the bar ("pinching" the joint into a distorted position under a load of weight); doing dips with the wrong bio-mechanical set-up; or, from all out heavy lifting without enough rest. This inflammation, if not dealt with can turn into a need for an operation on the AC joint. As soon as you feel a pinching feeling in the AC joint, stop and proceed to rest and ice each day for at least a week. For those who really inflame the Ac joint, there is an orthoscopic surgery that can be preformed; but, remember, every surgery has risks, and a smart bodybuilder never allows this joint, or any joint to get to the point where surgery is the only answer. (Some people actually respond better to heat; especially when it comes to tendinitis).

Elbows, Wrists, Knees, and Ankles

As stated, the circumference of any joint will determine the power and leverage advantage you will have in certain exercises. When evaluating yourself, look at the wrists and elbows and know that one and/or both of these joints could be small for your skeletal frame. Often times, wrist wraps help so as to allow for a straight line to the bar without weakness. Often, bodybuilders will use knee wraps to squat or leg press heavily. This is an idea that has been debated for decades. It really comes down to your own body and decision as to whether wraps are going to be of help to you. The problem with wrapping is that you could be damaging a joint and not knowing it; however, often wrapping prevents injuries, and thus one must try if necessary.

The elbow and wrist can easily be overworked, or worked disproportionately – causing inflammation and tendinitis. Again, stretching, light work and ice are common remedies; however with the elbow tendinitis, often it comes from using the ulna flexor (the inner belly of the forearm) too much and not working the radial (outside) area to keep the forearm balanced with strength. This is important to remember because almost everyone works the ulna flexor more because grabbing and squeezing the bar or dumbbell tends to work this area without working it directly. The radial area (the outside of the forearm) should be worked by doing reverse wrist curls; and reverse curls (with an e-z-curl bar).

Serious injuries to any joint can happen when using either too much weight; or poor form. Take a look at each joint to understand how they articulate. Remember, the standard home remedy for any injury is R.I.C.E.: Rest, ice, compression, elevation. Compression is done by wrapping the joint in ice with an ace-bandage. Elevation means to elevate the injury above the heart. This simple act will arrest the bodies' natural defense mechanisms of sending free radicals to the area in stress. The faster you use R.I.C.E., the faster you will recover from simple injuries.

Gloves, Straps, Hanging Boots, Etc.

Years ago, no one used gloves to work out; it was considered sort of a wimpy thing to do. However, people who have small hands, or a weak grip do benefit from wearing gloves when using weights for the upper body. If, however, you really have good size hands and want to build strength in your hands and forearms, skip wearing gloves and build up calluses and a hugely powerful handshake.

As with gloves, years ago if you were doing pull-ups or pull-downs, you did it until you lost your grip or fatigued the muscles. Often, the former comes before the later and thus I believe straps for these types of exercises do have advantages.

Other pieces of gear that have some logical use are gravitational boots; which allow the person to hang upside down from a pull-up bar and thus allowing the entire spine to relax in a position where I have seen people (including myself) relocate herniated discs, relax and help the lumbar area of the spine. It is difficult to totally relax while hanging upside down; however, in a short period of time you will get the hang of it.

Gym Balls and Weight Training

It has become a fad with trainers and some novice weight trainers to lift weights while lying on a ball. I have one word for this: STUPID. The idea of creating MMS is to put your body at a stable and leverage advantaged position. You cannot do that while jiggling all around on a big blue ball. No matter which "core" muscles you may be working, you are either going to injure yourself; or, simply not get MMS, which as I have explained leads to Maximum Muscle Hypertrophy.

This completes the training section of the book. For other questions about training and routine layouts, you may turn to Q&A and my training routine at the end of the book.

Let us now turn our attention inward, to what we eat, how we should eat, and what is the history of food consumption and how it either contributes to rapid aging; or, helps you age gracefully.

Notes:

Notes:

6 | Human Food Consumption

The Evolution of Human Food Consumption

Early ape-humans were hunter-gatherers. They ate whatever, whenever they could. During our early evolution three major but distinct groups of proto-humans were pushed out of the Jungles of Africa because of a geological change of weather patterns on that continent. These distinct groups of proto-humans took various routes of travel from their origins and thus took up various forms of eating according to what they found on their route out of Africa. One thing is for certain, without an ocean to divide this enormous land mass, these proto-humans spread over the entire area from Europe to China.

The group we are primarily interested in is the one that survived and would later become Homo sapiens, our ancestors. The other two major groups died off because they were what paleo-nutritionologists call "specialists." They tried to survive on a diet of wild roots and leaves. By remaining frugovours (fruit eaters) and/or folivoures (leaf eaters) they perished. Hunting to them was unheard of because they were surrounded by vegetation.

Homo sapiens became carnivorous omnivores and found their way around the world, continuing to grow both physically and mentally as they hunted, killed and ate wild animals, eating their catch raw for over a million years before learning the taste benefits of cooked meat although "raw" food is superior to cooked. They also gathered wild vegetables, roots, nuts, and berries. This all took great strength and effort, teamwork, raw speed and power to hunt down huge animals and find wild roots and berries and nuts – all scattered around the forests and jungles that Homo sapiens walked into. These human powerhouses became seasonally nomadic, constantly on the move doing daily tasks and tracking the herds of animals, often for hundreds of miles on foot in horrendous conditions. It also took great intelligence to coordinate the hunt, track, locate, and kill the animals. This innate intelligence is unique in all of mammalian evolution. The key here is that our ancestors survived because of this intelligence and because they hunted and ate wild game, gathered and ate wild vegetables, roots, nuts, seeds and berries.

The Change of The Guard in Evolution

Our ancestors participated in the aforementioned life style until somewhere between 10,000 – 2,000 years ago, depending on the location of the tribe. At this period in history, the world changed for humans in every conceivable way. Slowly, but surely the brain became so intelligent (because our earliest ancestors used their hands to crush the skulls of carcasses left behind by carnivores) and ate the brains of all types of animals and in those brains are loads of DHA and DEA – two important acids that are needed for outer cortex construction. In other words; we became "intelligent" because our earliest ancestors survived by eating the "leftovers" of a kill by another wild animal.

Those early ancestors used their fingers, their amazing hands (that they passed along to us with amazing dexterity) and smashed the skull of carcasses and ate the brains. This was the beginning of our "brain" as we know it today. Because of the development of our brains no other mammal on earth can do what we can do.

During the post Neo-Paleolithic, or animal and plant domestication era set evolution and human dietary habits on a new course, as you shall see. The six most commonly agreed upon areas in the world where this type of living had its origins are: The Fertile Crescent (8,500 B.C.), China (7,500 B.C.), Central and Southern Mexico (3,000 B.C.), Central America, the Andes of South America (3,000 B.C.), possibly the Amazon Basin (3,000 B.C.), and the eastern region of the United States (2,500 B.C.)

It is believed each of these areas above (with the exception of Europe and North America) began food production without influence from each other, using the indigenous plants and animals that were easiest to tame, coral, plant and domesticate. These were not simple matters and required creative intelligence that would rival any rocket scientist of today.

The Fundamentals of Ancient Plant Domestication

Of all the potential edible foliage in the world, only one percent is fit for human consumption. It took many thousands of years to know which plants could be domesticated for human consumption. Some groups domesticated earlier than others probably due to the respective availability of food. Once the natural supply of wild game, plants and fruits began to diminish within an area, an effort had to be made to find new ways of procuring food, usually this meant moving on to better hunting grounds and new forests where fruits, roots and berries would be more plentiful. At some point, depending on necessity, tribes realized that if they could raise one or two crops of edible plants it was much more efficient than wandering through the woods looking for wild vegetation. Observing events around them, such as the fact that melons grew from seeds in piles of animal feces may have helped early farmers (still hunter-gatherers) realize that not only could they grow fruit from seeds found in the fruit, but also that animal feces helped fertilize the crop's growth.

Early plant domestication would change the evolution of plants through the clever examination of very observant people who would one day be called "farmers." For example, wild almonds are deadly poisonous. The intensely bitter taste from an almond comes from amygdalin, which breaks down into the lethal gas cyanide. In the almond tree one or two trees out of thousands contains a genetic mutation that prevents it from producing amygdalin and the almonds from these trees are "sweet" edible almonds. However, birds and animals could and did eat these almonds putting the mutated trees at a disadvantage in evolutionary terms. Since the seeds from these trees were being eaten, there were not as many trees with the mutation reproduced. Thus the species remained intact as it had evolved – with poison fruit.

Early humans observed birds and other animals eating these sweet almonds and with their intelligence, powers of conjecture and newly found agrarian skills could plant and grow these mutated almond trees with the "sweet" nuts. Thus, the process of natural selection which would normally have exterminated a mutation of this type, had been interrupted by humans ability to selectively grow these mutated trees from seeds they had gathered thereby creating an entire crop of mutant plants.

Another clear example of humans altering the course of plant evolution can be understood by mapping the progression of the little green pea. In the wild, when the peas are ripe the pod explodes and peas are shot all around the outlying area to grow new plants. However, in 5% of the plants the pods do not explode. Normally, the peas from these defective plants would die entombed in their pods withering away in the sun. However, early on in our history humans took the seeds from these mutant pea plants and planted them so that the harvest of the peas would be easier and more efficient than scrambling in the dirt for each single pea from the exploding pod. Once again, human intervention saved a mutant plant from extinction and changed the course of evolution.

Wheat and barley, two of the most widely used crops in the world today, in their "wild" state drop their seeds when the stalk "shudders" in the wind. This "shuddering" ability is an evolutionary development to aid in the spread of the seeds. There are mutated plants on which the stalk does not shudder and thus the seeds stay on the plant. In the wild, this mutation would soon disappear because these seeds would not have the advantage of the seeds that get spread on the ground. However, humans once again observed this and saw the benefit of keeping the seeds on the stalk for harvesting and decided to plant and grow seeds from these mutated plants. Over thousands of years of this process, we now have wheat and barley fields entirely made up of the mutant plants.

Humans began eating a diet consisting of mutated plants and domesticated animals. They took the trees and plants that normally would have been wiped out by nature because they were defective and changed evolution by domesticating them. Clearly, this was the zenith of human creativity and yet, it was our intelligence that changed evolution and all the world's cultures forever.

The Fundamentals of Animal Domestication

There were only fourteen wild herbivores in the entire world that made it onto the domesticated list. Of those ancient fourteen, the "minor nine" are: Arabian camel, Bactrian camel, llama, donkey, reindeer, water buffalo, yak, banteng and gaur. The remaining "major five" are: cow, sheep, goat, pig and horse. Domesticated animals differ in many ways from their wild ancestors for two reasons.

1.) Human selection and breeding to get the "best" results has changed the form and shape of these animals to suit human tastes not nature's taste.

2.) Automatic evolutionary responses of animals to the artificial environment has altered the forces of natural selection to allow those animals who are better suited to such an environment to survive.

Domesticated animals have changed physiologically and organically; brains, muscles, and organs slowly atrophied, just as ours would over the upcoming millenniums.

With these changes has come a weakening of the domesticated animals that we eat. This adds to something that I go into later in the book as to the actual energy acquired from eating a cow that barely moves during its entire life and eating a wild deer or elk that never stops moving. Energy is a big part of food consumption although few nutritionists give it any thought beyond the protein, carbohydrate and fat make up of that particular animal. My belief is that the more "wild" the energy inside the animal's parasympathetic and autonomic nervous systems the more "energy" in the food. Energy cannot be seen. Remember, energy never disappears; it merely changes form. The energy from the Big Bang at the beginning of the Universe is what keeps this planet moving and keeps us all alive.

The Human Physiological Consequences of Food Production

The average Neo-Palaeolithian male was 6′ tall, while the average female was 5′6″ tall. They were classically mesomorphic (muscular and lean) with an amazing balance of slow and fast twitch muscle fibers which allowed for both quick explosive strength and the ability to run long distances. This phenomenal athletic ability was without question the result of thousands of years of hunter-gatherer culture – exercising daily, eating wild meat, and wild roots, vegetables, nuts, fruits and seeds.

With the advent of plant and animal domestication the human skeleton started shrinking approximately .75 of an inch for each millennium. By the Middle Ages, the average European male, direct descendant of the once super-athletic Upper Palaeolithians, was approximately 5'5" and had the physique of a modern-day couch potato. A loss of six inches in nine thousand years! How did this happen? The decrease in wild, dense animal protein, an increase in mutant grain consumption, an increase in saturated fat due to the higher levels found in sedentary domesticated animals, and the steady loss of vigorous physical activity all contributed to this loss of stature.

Conclusions About Agrarianism

Two very important conclusions can be drawn from studying these historical events pertaining to food production which also had a huge bearing on the way we eat and live today as well as how the world has been shaped religiously and geo-political-ly.

1.) The introduction of grains as a primary food source weakened the human physiology to a large degree. (Remember these were "whole" grains, not the pulverized, refined grains that many eat today). This is one of the many reasons I believe in eliminating all refined foods and, for some, all grains. This is also good enough evidence for me to choose to eat plenty of animal protein provided it's clean of drugs and low in saturated fat.

2.) Agrarianism and food producing would lead us into our three modern nutritional dilemmas:

a) The pancreas is being overwhelmed with refined carbohydrates (pulverized flour products), and our bodies are aging faster because of the increased insulin levels needed to store these refined forms of glucose. Increased insulin leads to insulin resistance, which leads to a host of problems. Much more on this later.

b) We have become so reliant on food-production, we are at the mercy of farmers who use antibiotics, steroids, growth hormones to either fatten the beef, or keep the animals from spreading germs and bacteria within their horribly confined living-quarters before being slaughtered. Although the government tries to regulate this they are very lenient with farmers because the farmer has a very narrow margin of profit. When choosing meats, try to buy meat that is raised "free range" and naturally.

c) The energy of a domesticated plant such as wheat, or that of a sedentary cow is weak and counter-evolutionary. On top of that, we have been exposed to animal tissue that has been not only genetically altered but, in the past fifty years at least, chemically altered. There can be no doubt that eating these genetically and chemically altered species has not only changed our physiology, but also changed our "energy."

Even though today Americans and Europeans are bigger and stronger than anytime since the neo-Paleolithic era, mostly because of the fact that we all eat adequate supplies of protein, the amount of body fat on a contemporary person has increased threefold because of total caloric increase, especially high-glycemic, refined carbohydrates and higher saturated fat in live-stock. The more refined processed food we eat as postmodern humans, the further away from true evolutionary physiology and dynamic energy we will go. I have no doubt about this.

It seems to me there is an actual physiological and psychological change that takes place when eating something directly from a tree or the ground and food taken from animals that lived "wild", compared to something that has been made synthetically. What history teaches us, and what science tells us today, is what we should eat and how and why we age from what we eat.

Notes:

Notes:

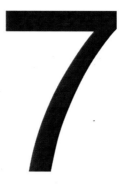

Why & How We Age: An Organic Explanation

The Universal Biological Markers of Aging

This section of Burke's Law focuses on diet and aging and how much of your appearance and aging processes are influenced by what you eat. By giving you this scientific information, it is my hope that you will understand that the combination of an anti-aging diet and a very high-tech type of workout routine, as outlined previously in the book, will help you in reaching your potential for longevity and building a fabulous body. Let us begin by examining how the aging process works.

Chapter Sixteen:
The Universal Biological Markers of Aging

First let us establish exactly what, a "biological marker" is. "Biological markers" are both not only measurable and quantifiable, but also universal. They can be tracked throughout human history, and observed over time. They cross all ethnic, racial, and gender barriers. For example, the fact that systolic blood pressure tends to rise as we age, regardless of ethnicity, race, or gender, is a biological marker.

There are four biological markers that increase with age, and six that decrease with age.

In contemplating this chart, one can quickly see that there is an interesting correlation between what increases with age and what decreases. The increase in one's insulin resistance, for example, leads to a greater chance for developing glucose intolerance. As cells become resistant to insulin, there are higher levels of glucose remaining in the blood. Likewise, a person's decreased aerobic capacity means that the heart must work that much harder to move the blood into outlying areas, thereby paving the way for chronic high systolic blood pressure to develop. As more insulin is secreted due to high-glycemic carbohydrates and/or overeating, cells become more resistant and one

Age Related Biological Markers	
Markers That _Increase_ With Age	**Markers That _Decrease_ With Age**
Insulin Resistance	Glucose Intolerance
Systolic Blood Pressure	Aerobic Capacity
Percentage of Body Fat	Muscle Mass
Lipid Ratios	Strength
	Temperature Regulation
	Immune Function

begins to store higher levels of adipose tissue or body fat. This, in turn, increases LDL (low density lipoprotein) levels, and almost simultaneously increases the chance for arterial sclerosis and other coronary problems. These conditions are of special concern for people who have a family history of heart disease. Further, the amount of body fat that a person carries is directly related to how much insulin they produce and how little lean muscle mass they have. The lower one's percentage of lean muscle mass, the less support one's skeleton enjoys, and therefore a limiting of functionality will ultimately ensue. Limited functionality, in turn, gives way to a loss of strength, which then leads to a decrease in growth hormone production (See Graphic D, page 154), the component needed for muscle building. Increased levels of stored body fat also slow the tissue repair process. If the tissue repair process takes too long, muscles risk atrophying from non-use, and lipid ratios will begin to rise. With a rise in lipid ratios, temperature regulation systems begin to fail, and the body's immune functions are ultimately compromised. Each of the body's other systems will begin to fail, too, and the negative aspects of the aging process become readily apparent.

Luckily, all of these aging processes are reversible, if you are willing to watch your diet and by participating in a moderate workout program. Each of these biological markers is influenced by how and what we eat, how we use our bodies for exercise and/or motion, and to some degree, how well we regulate our emotions. Immortality remains out of the question, but careful attention to diet and exercise will help us to maintain our health longer and to live a more vital life.

From these observations, we can deduce that there are four known primary mechanisms that affect these biological markers. According to a theory postulated by Bernard Streheler in the late 1980's, an aging mechanism explains why we experience a loss in physiological function over time. This same mechanism must also explain why this loss is gradual, and why the losses are intrinsic.

Scientific Theories on Aging

There are many schools of thought regarding the mechanisms of aging. One theory proposes that aging is programmed in our DNA. Meaning, there is literally a clock ticking, and when the programmed hour arrives, you die. Russian aging expert Vladimir Dilman first proposed this theory, asserting that the internal "clock" could be found in the brain's hypothalamus, the home of the endocrine system, the part of the brain considered the "control-central" for hormonal communication.

The hypothalamus is influenced by feedback loops that respond to hormonal levels. All of the body's physiological systems are affected by hormones, therefore this theory not only makes good scientific sense, it also gives us an opportunity to consider the possibility of a definite link between hormonal communication and aging. If this is true, we can assume that how we choose to eat and exercise can certainly affect our overall health and longevity, given that diet and exercise have such a profound affect on the endocrine system.

An alternative theory on aging, put forth by Robert Sapolsky of Stanford University, focuses on the glucocorticoid cascade mechanism. Sapolsky argues that, as levels of the corticosteroid cortisol are released by the adrenal glands during times of physical, emotional, or endocrine [8] stress, the body begins to store the cortisol, which over time leads to the death of neurons within the brain. As these neurons die or are damaged, the feedback message is also damaged, which leads to a release of even greater amounts of cortisol into the bloodstream. A catch-22 develops, and, the autocrine [9] and endocrine systems fail. Death is not too far behind. As anyone who has ever taken any type of corticosteroid knows, it doesn't take these powerful hormones much time to affect nearly all aspects of the body.

Eicosonoid production (the underlying autocrine hormone that regulates not only the heart rate, but also the entire immune system) is also affected by the introduction of excess corticosteroids. Nevertheless, eicosonoids are, historically, a part of the oldest hormonal system of the body (the autocrine system). They are, as Dr. Barry Sears, of "The Zone" plan likes to call them, "the molecular glue that holds all the body's systems together."

As an extreme example of a cascading mechanistic failure brought on by hormone levels can be found in the life of the Pacific salmon. After swimming against heavy currents for several weeks, the salmon reaches his desired mating destination, only to mate and die within days. How and why, you might ask? The relentless struggle against the current leaves the salmon's body inundated with the stress hormone cortisol. Cortisol levels are too high, and all of his systems then fail. Elevated cortisol levels are responsible for all kinds of maladies in humans and animals alike, such as stroke, cancer, and heart disease. You must keep this in mind as you begin working out over long and frequent periods. Working out inherently subjects the body to stress – stress produces cortisol, therefore I have developed a way to train that is focused on short, intense workouts that also incorporate mild cardiovascular work, such as brisk walking and mild and frequent stretching. Combined, these elements will help lower your cortisol production levels.

Another identifiable mechanism of aging has been identified through DNA research focused on the tail-like fragments attached to the tips of chromosomes. These fragments are called telomeres. Each time a new cell division occurs, the telomere is shortened slightly. After so many divisions, the telomere is depleted, and the cell dies. Scientists have determined that, in order to fight the forces of aging, cell division should be kept to a minimum. How can we achieve this? Let us see.

The on/off process of DNA replication is controlled by the body's production of what are known as "growth factors." Insulin, which functions primarily as a storage hormone, is one of the most powerful growth factors of all. Bodybuilders who take insulin and growth factor-1 age anywhere from two to five times more quickly than normal, depending on how much sugar they eat and how much cortisol they produce. Moderate exercise, you will be pleased to learn, can offset the negative effects of insulin and growth factor production. Moderate levels of exercise only produce the slightest amounts of cortisol. Also, glucose uptake during exercise is a non insulin-driven event. That is to say, blood sugar and insulin levels are both decreased and normalized by regular, moderate exercise.

The FInal Word on Insulin

The more insulin you produce, the more your cells are encouraged to grow. The more cell growth you experience, the more protein your body requires. The more protein you require, the more cell growth you will achieve, and therefore you will deplete an increasing number of telomeres. Therefore, we can conclude that there is a very fine line between producing enough insulin to store nutrients in cells and producing too much insulin to maintain regular health. Also, excessive amounts of exercise will lead to excessive cell growth (division), and an unnecessary depletion of telomeres.

Free Radicals and Anti-Oxidants

In the 1950's, Denham Harman developed an interesting theory on aging, the free radical concept of disease. Harman believed that aging was a consequence of an overproduction of free radicals, atoms or molecules with an unpaired electron.

The air that we breathe is, according to scientists, comprised of relatively inert gassy molecules. Unless the body extracts an electron from an oxygen atom (O2) to form a free radical, it cannot react with other molecules to maintain the constantly vigorous processes that control the body and give us life. Once the electron is extracted, an oxygen free radical, forms, and aerobic life can begin. During the first three billion years on this planet, life was anaerobic, the photosynthetic process had not yet begun, and the single-celled microorganisms present on Earth did not require oxygen. With the emergence of photosynthetic organisms approximately 3.5 to 2.75 billion years ago, oxygen began accumulating in the atmosphere and aerobic organisms developed to take advantage of this new oxygen-rich environment.

These early aerobic organisms devised ways to convert oxygen into water, and in turn, used the extraction process to create energy. Remember this, for this concept is very much tied into ATP production and the forces that govern muscles during weight training and other short-term anaerobic exercises. As you know, the body constantly produces ATP to provide for short bursts of energy. To make this ATP, you must first produce an oxygen free radical. Under normal circumstances, a person only has enough ATP to last for about 10 seconds before the body must make more – which requires more free radical production. This is why Burke's Law advocates efforts to increase your ATP production capacity. As ATP is used, lactic acid is released into the fatigued muscle, thus inhibiting its continued use. From a biological standpoint, training with weights in order to build muscle and increase strength should be done in short bursts of all-out effort, allowing just enough resting between sets for the body to make more ATP. Any other training method will not be as effective, and borders on aerobic training, which does not build muscle or strength as effectively as anaerobic work.

Remember, the body must produce ATP from free radicals; unfortunately, approximately 6% of all free radicals produced will escape to become "rogue" free radicals. Those that roam free remain unpaired, and naturally begin looking for a mate. They seek out neighboring molecules in the body, and attach themselves in an effort to become "whole." If this neighbor happens to be protein, DNA, or fat, this new molecule in turn becomes a new free radical.

The natural opponents of free radicals are anti-oxidants. Leading anti-oxidants include vitamins A, C, and E, selenium, and alpha lipoic acid. These vitamins are called anti-oxidants because they sacrifice themselves in an effort to stop this rogue free-radical propagation, which, if left unchecked, will lead to the oxidization and death of cells. Vitamins don't, of course, stop aging or guarantee health, but they certainly do a great deal to help slow this natural degenerative process. An easy way to visualize the oxidization process is to think of a piece of metal that has been exposed to water and the elements. Rust develops, and small areas are destroyed. This is exactly what happens to cells when free radicals are made. Consequently, you should avoid overeating and over-exercising, in an effort to reduce free radical formation and cell death. If cellular defense enzymes and antioxidants, such as superoxide dimutase (SOD), [10] are not present or successfully made, the newly formed free radicals can cross-link with other free radicals to form polymerized products. Polymerized products can be a serious problem because they contribute to rapid cellular degeneration and aging.

Supplementing your diet with essential fatty acids such as Omega-3 is vital for your health. These fats, however, are easily removed by oxygen free radicals, thus leaving behind a new free radical to react with oxygen to form a peralkoxy free radical. These new, more stable free radicals can inflict serious damage on cells as they seek out new electrons to strip. Once an essential fatty acid has been stripped and/or oxidized, it can no longer carry out its vital function of forming eicosonoids, the autocrine hormones that are the cellular foundation of the body's functions. When you supplement your diet with these essential fatty acids, such as Omega-3, you are providing a valuable defense against the rogue free radicals that propel the aging process.

Returning for a moment to the so-called "rogue" free radicals: when a free radical attacks a DNA molecule, a genetic mutation occurs that, if unchecked, will be perpetuated during subsequent replication cycles. In other words, these damaged cells will not contain healthy DNA blueprints, and the cells become prone to further mutation or attack, leading them to become cancerous.

As you can see, the more free radicals your body produces, the more rogue free radicals escape and attack the vital elements of your body. In descending order, food digestion, high levels of stress and the subsequent release of cortisol, and excessive amounts of exercise bring about free radical production. Digestion, by far, produces the most free radicals. Overeating, then, leads to an entirely avoidable increase in free radical production. Additionally, the more insulin-producing carbohydrates in your meals, the more energy digestion will require, and, of course, more free radicals will be produced.

Simply put, calories in food must be turned into a form of energy that the body can use; however to form this fuel from food, it produces free radicals. Perhaps as much of 90% of all the free radicals you will make in your lifetime will come as a result of the digestive process. Later in this chapter I will help you calculate how much food you should consume at each meal, so as to guarantee adequate energy levels while still guarding against excessive free radical production.

After digestion, the primary way free radicals are generated is through the immune system. White blood cells are formed by free radicals in order to attack foreign invaders. Therefore, people with high, or chronically low, white blood cell counts often feel tired and rundown. Their immune systems are working overtime to produce white blood cells to fight off bacteria or a virus.

In addition to the three mechanisms of aging we have already discussed, increased cortisol, insulin, and free radical levels, there is one additional mechanism of aging remaining, the formation of advanced glycocylated end-products (AGEs).

AGEs are the most recently discovered of the mechanisms of aging, and are responsible for the cross-linking of glucose (carbohydrates) and protein. AGEs have a very strong impact on aging and the development of degenerative illnesses. Any time there are elevated levels of glucose in the bloodstream, it is likely that cross-linking will occur. That is to say, every time you overeat, especially if you have indulged in high-glycemic carbohydrates, cross-linking will occur, thereby doubling the speed of your aging process.

In addition to speeding the aging process, elevated glucose levels also result in damage to the glucose-sensitive region of the hypothalamus known as the ventromedial nucleus. This area of the hypothalamus is responsible for sending messages to the pancreas telling it when and how much insulin to secrete. Glucose-induced damage impairs this feedback system, and results in the pancreas overproducing insulin. Insulin resistance is the natural consequence of this, as is the onset of Type II diabetes.

Now that we have examined at what speeds the aging process, let us try to figure out how to slow it down.

Relevant Charts and Graphics

Graphic A

The interesting markers of biological aging and how they influence each other.

Graphic B

The Glucagon/Insulin Axis. Take note of the proper hormonal balance needed to keep the body in homeostasis. This "see-saw" battle is won or lost by the food choices outlined in this chapter.

Graphic C

Cyclic AMP is a "messenger" that decodes cell membranes to allow nutrients and hormones into cells and organs. It is also directly influenced by the food eaten at each meal. Without this "second messenger," hormones cannot reach target cells and organs.

Graphic D

The release of Growth hormone and what inhibits it/and/or promotes its release.

Graphic E

The complicated release of the hormone Testosterone.

Graphic F

The evolution of hormonal communication from single cell; to our amazingly complex trilogy hormonal system.

Graphic G

What roles various types of fats play in hormonal replication and communication.

Graphic H

Biological Mechanisms Active During and After Exercise.

A.

Biological Markers of Human Aging

MARKERS THAT INCREASE
- Insulin Resistance
- Systolic Blood Pressure
- Percentage of Body Fat
- Lipid Ratios

MARKERS THAT DECREASE
- Glucose Tolerance
- Aerobic Capacity
- Muscle Mass
- Strength
- Temperature Regulation
- Immune Function

UNDERSTOOD MECHANISMS BEHIND BIOLOGICAL MARKERS
1.) Excess Insulin
2.) Excess Blood-Glucose
3.) Excess Free-Radicals
4.) Excess Cortisol

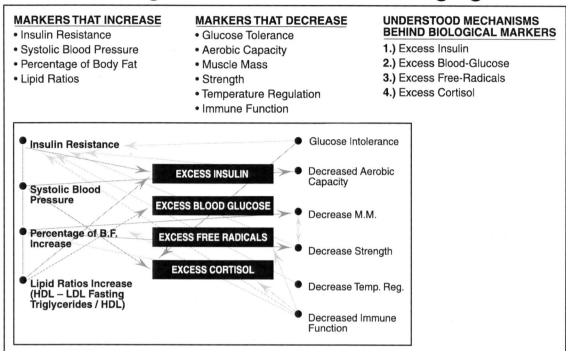

B.

Glucagon / Insulin Axis

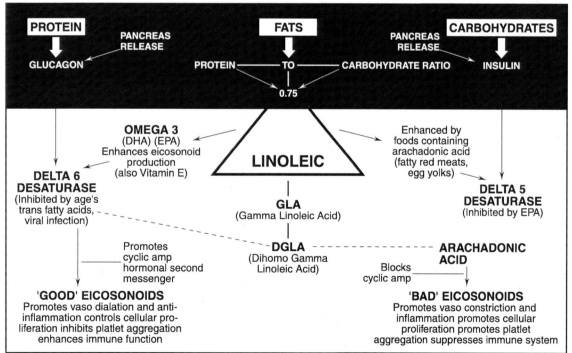

C.   # Cyclic Amp

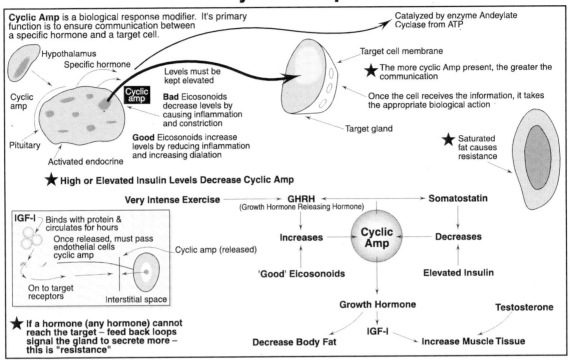

Cyclic Amp is a biological response modifier. It's primary function is to ensure communication between a specific hormone and a target cell.

Catalyzed by enzyme Andeylate Cyclase from ATP

Hypothalamus
Specific hormone
Levels must be kept elevated

Cyclic amp

Cyclic amp

Bad Eicosonoids decrease levels by causing inflammation and constriction

Good Eicosonoids increase levels by reducing inflammation and increasing dialation

Pituitary

Activated endocrine

Target cell membrane

★ The more cyclic Amp present, the greater the communication

Once the cell receives the information, it takes the appropriate biological action

Target gland

★ Saturated fat causes resistance

★ High or Elevated Insulin Levels Decrease Cyclic Amp

Very Intense Exercise → **GHRH** ← **Somatostatin**
(Growth Hormone Releasing Hormone)

IGF-I Binds with protein & circulates for hours
Once released, must pass endothelial cells cyclic amp

Cyclic amp (released)

On to target receptors

Interstitial space

Increases   **Cyclic Amp**   **Decreases**

'Good' Eicosonoids   Elevated Insulin

Growth Hormone   Testosterone

★ If a hormone (any hormone) cannot reach the target — feed back loops signal the gland to secrete more — this is "resistance"

Decrease Body Fat   IGF-I   Increase Muscle Tissue

D.   # Release of Polypeptide Hormone GH. Half-Life 5-6 Mins.

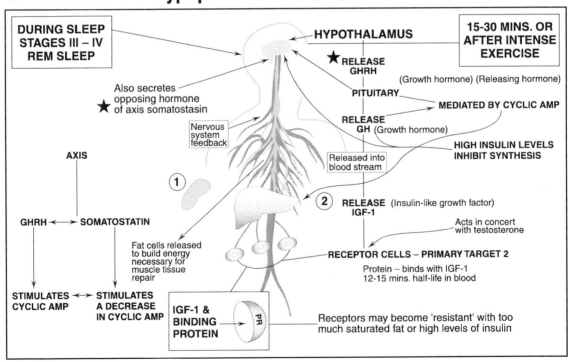

DURING SLEEP STAGES III – IV REM SLEEP

HYPOTHALAMUS

15-30 MINS. OR AFTER INTENSE EXERCISE

Also secretes opposing hormone ★ of axis somatostasin

★ **RELEASE GHRH**

(Growth hormone) (Releasing hormone)

PITUITARY

MEDIATED BY CYCLIC AMP

Nervous system feedback

RELEASE GH (Growth hormone)

HIGH INSULIN LEVELS INHIBIT SYNTHESIS

Released into blood stream

AXIS

①

② **RELEASE** (Insulin-like growth factor) **IGF-1**

Acts in concert with testosterone

GHRH ←→ SOMATOSTATIN

Fat cells released to build energy necessary for muscle tissue repair

RECEPTOR CELLS – PRIMARY TARGET 2

Protein – binds with IGF-1 12-15 mins. half-life in blood

STIMULATES ←→ STIMULATES
CYCLIC AMP   A DECREASE IN CYCLIC AMP

IGF-1 & BINDING PROTEIN

PR

Receptors may become 'resistant' with too much saturated fat or high levels of insulin

158

E.

Testosterone

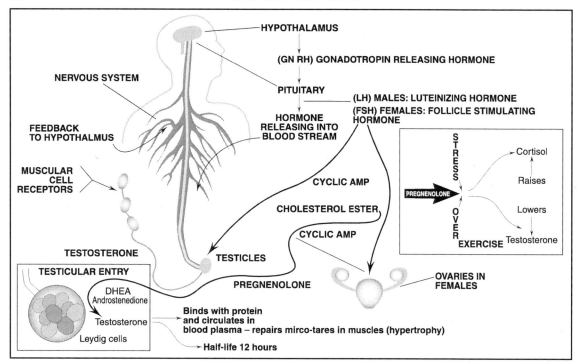

HYPOTHALAMUS

(GN RH) GONADOTROPIN RELEASING HORMONE

NERVOUS SYSTEM

PITUITARY

(LH) MALES: LUTEINIZING HORMONE
(FSH) FEMALES: FOLLICLE STIMULATING HORMONE

FEEDBACK
TO HYPOTHALMUS

HORMONE
RELEASING INTO
BLOOD STREAM

MUSCULAR
CELL
RECEPTORS

CYCLIC AMP

CHOLESTEROL ESTER

STRESS OVER EXERCISE

Cortisol

Raises

PREGNENOLONE

Lowers

Testosterone

CYCLIC AMP

TESTOSTERONE

TESTICLES

OVARIES IN
FEMALES

TESTICULAR ENTRY

PREGNENOLONE

DHEA
Androstenedione

Testosterone

Leydig cells

**Binds with protein
and circulates in
blood plasma – repairs mirco-tares in muscles (hypertrophy)**

Half-life 12 hours

F.

Basic Hormonal Communication

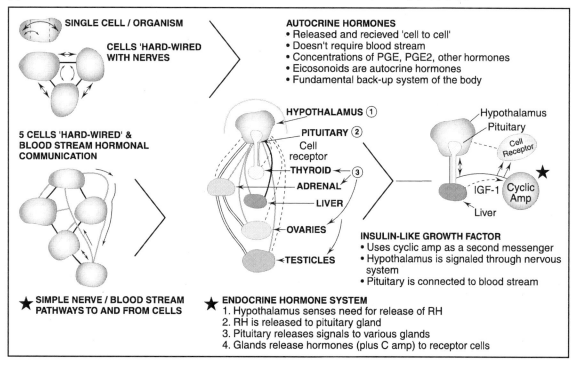

SINGLE CELL / ORGANISM

CELLS 'HARD-WIRED
WITH NERVES

AUTOCRINE HORMONES
• Released and recieved 'cell to cell'
• Doesn't require blood stream
• Concentrations of PGE, PGE2, other hormones
• Eicosonoids are autocrine hormones
• Fundamental back-up system of the body

5 CELLS 'HARD-WIRED' &
BLOOD STREAM HORMONAL
COMMUNICATION

HYPOTHALAMUS ①

Hypothalamus
Pituitary

PITUITARY ②

Cell
receptor

Cell
Receptor

THYROID ← ③

ADRENAL

IGF-1

Cyclic
Amp

LIVER

Liver

OVARIES

TESTICLES

INSULIN-LIKE GROWTH FACTOR
• Uses cyclic amp as a second messenger
• Hypothalamus is signaled through nervous
  system
• Pituitary is connected to blood stream

★ **SIMPLE NERVE / BLOOD STREAM
PATHWAYS TO AND FROM CELLS**

★ **ENDOCRINE HORMONE SYSTEM**
1. Hypothalamus senses need for release of RH
2. RH is released to pituitary gland
3. Pituitary releases signals to various glands
4. Glands release hormones (plus C amp) to receptor cells

G. **Fats**

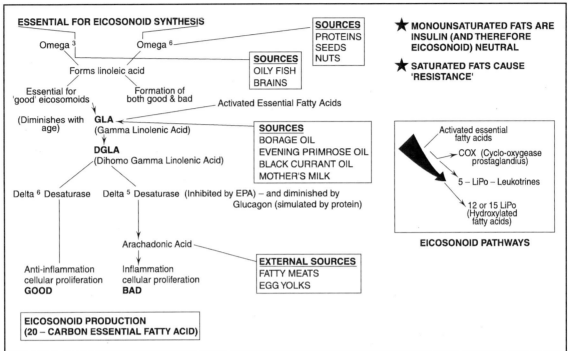

ESSENTIAL FOR EICOSONOID SYNTHESIS

Omega 3   Omega 6

SOURCES
PROTEINS
SEEDS
NUTS

Forms linoleic acid

SOURCES
OILY FISH
BRAINS

Essential for 'good' eicosomoids   Formation of both good & bad

Activated Essential Fatty Acids

(Diminishes with age)   **GLA**
(Gamma Linolenic Acid)

DGLA
(Dihomo Gamma Linolenic Acid)

SOURCES
BORAGE OIL
EVENING PRIMROSE OIL
BLACK CURRANT OIL
MOTHER'S MILK

★ MONOUNSATURATED FATS ARE INSULIN (AND THEREFORE EICOSONOID) NEUTRAL

★ SATURATED FATS CAUSE 'RESISTANCE'

Delta 6 Desaturase   Delta 5 Desaturase (Inhibited by EPA) – and diminished by Glucagon (simulated by protein)

Arachadonic Acid

EXTERNAL SOURCES
FATTY MEATS
EGG YOLKS

Anti-inflammation cellular proliferation **GOOD**

Inflammation cellular proliferation **BAD**

**EICOSONOID PRODUCTION
(20 – CARBON ESSENTIAL FATTY ACID)**

Activated essential fatty acids
COX (Cyclo-oxygease prostaglandius)
5 – LiPo – Leukotrines
12 or 15 LiPo (Hydroxylated fatty acids)

EICOSONOID PATHWAYS

H. **Biological Mechanisms Active During & After Exercise**

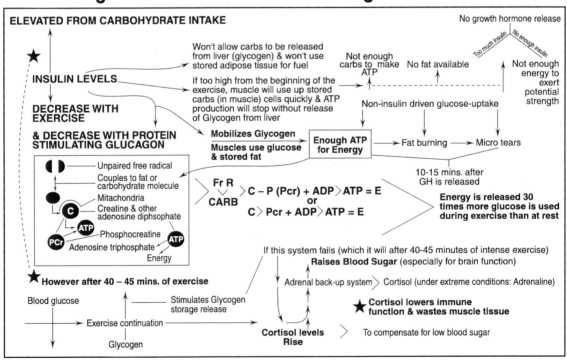

ELEVATED FROM CARBOHYDRATE INTAKE

No growth hormone release

★

INSULIN LEVELS

DECREASE WITH EXERCISE

& DECREASE WITH PROTEIN STIMULATING GLUCAGON

Won't allow carbs to be released from liver (glycogen) & won't use stored adipose tissue for fuel

If too high from the beginning of the exercise, muscle will use up stored carbs (in muscle) cells quickly & ATP production will stop without release of Glycogen from liver

Not enough carbs to make ATP

No fat available

Too much insulin   No enough insulin

Not enough energy to exert potential strength

Mobilizes Glycogen

Muscles use glucose & stored fat

Enough ATP for Energy

Non-insulin driven glucose-uptake

Fat burning → Micro tears

10-15 mins. after GH is released

Unpaired free radical
Couples to fat or carbohydrate molecule
Mitachondria
Creatine & other adenosine diphsophate
Phosphocreatine
Adenosine triphosphate
Energy

Fr R
CARB

$$C - P \ (Pcr) + ADP \rangle ATP = E$$
or
$$C \rangle Pcr + ADP \rangle ATP = E$$

Energy is released 30 times more glucose is used during exercise than at rest

★ **However after 40 – 45 mins. of exercise**

If this system fails (which it will after 40-45 minutes of intense exercise)
Raises Blood Sugar (especially for brain function)

Adrenal back-up system ⟩ Cortisol (under extreme conditions: Adrenaline)

Blood glucose

Stimulates Glycogen storage release

Exercise continuation

Glycogen

★ **Cortisol lowers immune function & wastes muscle tissue**

Cortisol levels Rise ⟩ To compensate for low blood sugar

Notes:

Notes:

8

Dieting for Health, Longevity & Muscle Building

- How Your Diet Affects the Mechanisms of Aging

Chapter Seventeen: How Your Diet Affects the Mechanisms of Aging

As the previous chapter illustrated, there are four primary causes of aging:

1.) Increased levels of cortisol

2.) Excessive insulin levels

3.) Excess free radicals

4.) Excess glucose

This chapter will show you how best to regulate these four occurrences. First, let us turn our attention to excess insulin production, as a discussion of insulin levels will lead naturally to examinations of glucose and cortisol levels.

In spite of many peoples' assumptions that insulin has something to do with sugar (which it does), it is primarily a storage hormone. Insulin stores nutrients within cells. You must have adequate insulin levels, in order to ensure proper feeding of your cells. Without it, they would suffer death. However, too much insulin speeds up aging and brings about death more quickly than almost any other biological process.

Excess insulin is produced when target cells no longer allow the insulin to store nutrients within the cell. When this happens, high glucose levels remain in the blood, and a feedback signal is sent to the hypothalamus, which in turn instructs the pancreas to secrete more insulin. At the same time, the affected cells begin to harden and become more rigid with each secretion of insulin, so the insulin begins to loose its ability to penetrate cells and store nutrients. Glucose levels remain high (potentially damaging brain cells and nerves), because penetration into cells is nearly impossible, and in response to this, if the (insulin and other hormone) resistance becomes bad enough, the adrenal glands begin trying to regulate blood glucose with cortisol. The cells that remain impenetrable, soon block the absorption of other hormones, and cell death begins.

The origins of age-related insulin resistance can be found by examining how our ancestors regulated their food consumption. Millions of years ago, humans did not eat "three square meals a day." Rather, starvation or deprivation conditions were the rule of the day. As a result, the pancreas was not called upon to secrete insulin several times per day, as it is in modern Western culture. Insulin was able to store nutrients in cells, and excess calories went to adipose tissue, better known as body fat. This stored body fat was used later as much-needed fuel for hunting and, crucially, as an aid in body temperature regulation. It is also important to note here that the insulin produced by our ancestors was not called upon to process the dense carbohydrates so commonly found in refined foods many of us eat today.

Our bodies have an amazing ability to turn stored fats into fuel, provided there are not high levels of glucose or insulin in the bloodstream. For this reason alone, carbohydrates should be kept in balance with protein, since protein's pancreatic response, glucagon [11], can counteract elevated levels of insulin in the blood. This is the notion upon which Barry Sears; founder of the popular "Zone" diet has based his entire life's work. In my opinion, this is the most logical way one can choose to eat. Having said that, I do not agree with Barry on every point in his first book. In his first book he allowed one to use refined foods so long as their glucagon/insulin axis was balanced. I do not believe in eating any refined foods for a variety of reasons, such as, they are like drugs and are hard to stop eating; they tend to be useless calories for the body; and, the body can become "allergic" or sensitive to refined foods. How would you like to be allergic to a refined food and you have a hard time taking it out of your diet because you are addicted to it? This addiction is similar to drug addiction; however, the "detoxing" of that food usually will only take two weeks. It is not a pleasant two weeks, but it is necessary for health and longevity.

Carbohydrates

Insulin resistance, such as that which accompanies Type II diabetes, occurs when, over a course of many years, a person who can either be predisposed or not – it really does not matter – takes in too many calories, and/or too many high-glycemic carbohydrates at each meal. Their cells become hardened and cannot absorb the nutrients that insulin is designed to put into the cells.

High-glycemic carbohydrates [12] are those carbohydrates that induce the pancreas to secrete excessive amounts of insulin in order to store the condensed and relative refined caloric content of the carbohydrate. They are termed "condensed," because, the more a carbohydrate is refined the more condensed it becomes, and the higher its glycemic factor. High glycemic factor carbohydrates require more insulin for storage. Three other nutritional factors also influence insulin and the glycemic index rankings of carbohydrates. They are: (1) the amount of roughage in the carbohydrate (which influences its absorption rate and the rate of pancreal insulin excretion); (2) the amount of fat taken in with the carbohydrate, which slows the absorption rate down; and (3) the amount of protein absorbed, which influences glucagon, and balances the insulin-related hormonal response of the pancreas. Each of these factors slow insulin's release into the bloodstream and can help protect you against premature aging, hypoglycemia, Type II diabetes, and the habitual storage of body fat. Be warned, however, saturated fat, that fat derived from domesticated animal products, can both increase insulin resistance and elevate LDL, or "bad" cholesterol. Most people with "Type II" Diabetes have insulin resistance as their main cause of high blood glucose.

High-glycemic carbohydrates are primarily found in foods made from refined grain products. A "refined" food is any food that has been altered from its original state. This even includes fruits dehydrated by the sun, such as raisins, and other dried fruits. They are considered high-glycemic carbohydrates because their nutritional make-up is, close if not equal to the simplicity and density of table sugar. Almost all breads and pastas, and all dehydrated foods, are also high on the glycemic index. "Why are they there?" You might wonder. These foods have high glycemic levels because the roughage and/or water naturally found within them has been removed, condensing them in such a way that the body overacts to their refinement. Our bodies did not evolve by eating foods such as these, but rather our ancestors focused on killing and gathering whole wild foods. The unnatural nature of a refined food-based diet is borne out in the realization that approximately one third of the population of the Unites States is presently, or will become, diabetic. Additionally, one third of all Americans will die from heart disease that will be directly relative to their insulin output, i.e., their eventual Type II diabetes. Approximately 15% of Americans will develop cancers brought on by cortisol and insulin problems. We have the ability to organically live to be 120 years old. Most won't because of these very problems we have created with an abundance of refined food, and high levels of stress with little knowledge of how to lower cortisol.

Raw Foods & DNA

Since our early ancestors ate nearly everything raw and wild, I would like you to understand the importance of this through modern science that shows the destructive nature of processed, cooked, or worst of all, micro-waved food.

The Role of Exercise and Raw and Wild Foods in Knocking Out Peroxynitrate

Peroxynitrite is a killer of cells; however, when ATP is generated, CO_2 is created as a by-product. CO_2 is a scavenger of peroxynitrite. The more you can create ATP (without producing cortisol), the longer your cells will allow penetration of hormones, macro/micro nutrients; and the more CO_2 you will make to scavenge for this killer nitrite. This means that your weight training workouts should be short, moderate with weights used and intense. If, for example, you workout too light or too fast, you will be using oxygen as fuel and therefore not utilizing ATP. On the other hand, if you workout too heavy and/or too long, you will produce cortisol which is an immune suppressant and can cause hypothalamus-pituitary-adrenal axis problems.

The other way to increase CO_2 and scavenge this cell killing nitrite is to make uric acid. Although it is not good to have too much uric acid, it is important to make it each day - throughout the day. Uric Acid is made from RNA and DNA metabolism that is produced both endogenously (withing the body) and exogenously (outside the body). There are certain foods that you can eat to produce your own endogenous RNA and DNA for uric acid production, which scavenges the cell killing peroxynitrite.

Exogenously driven, raw meat and fish are the greatest producers of RNA and DNA metabolism. Simply put, if you can eat good Sushi and get your hands on wild raw meat (that is safe), you can create superior DNA and RNA metabolism, which helps in the process of scavenging peroxynitrite and keeping cellular integrity. (Although RNA and DNA are constantly dying and being born, if you can contribute to the metabolic portion of this process you will make uric acid, which in turn will make more CO_2 and kill more peroxynitrite).

Now, if you don't like raw fish or (can't eat) raw meats, next on the list are raw vegetables in the form of (juicing); which should be limited to about 4-6 oz per day. Also, farm raised eggs, raw milk, raw cheese, raw butter are all filled with properties to help RNA and DNA metabolism.

The other new product on the market that helps this process is called Undenaturated Whey Protein. This is a product that has been changed molecularly from the standard whey protein to help with regulating what is called the Glutathione pathway. All of these foods help make uric acid, contribute to superior RNA and DNA metabolism and CO_2; which ultimately scavenges for peroxynitrite.

A simple way to think of this is that raw is better than cooked; young is better than old (thus the egg and raw milk); and unprocessed is better than processed. If you want to absolutely destroy all of the RNA and DNA metabolic qualities of any food, microwave your food - it will become nothing but empty calories.

So, before running around and buying every new diet book that comes along, learn from our ancestors and from modern science. Raw foods digest much easier and keep waste material moving out of the body all the time. Think about it: raw and unprocessed and it's good for you - can't be more simple that that.

Refined Vs. "Whole" Foods

Because they have been refined, once in the body, foods that have been altered induce the pancreas to respond with an abundance of insulin, oftentimes driving blood-glucose levels down, in an attempt to store the dense molecules in cells and/or body fat. While some people can tolerate these foods relatively well due to a naturally buffered pancreatic response [13], most people will eventually develop insulin-related problems. No matter who you are, the more insulin you make, the greater and faster the potential for cellular deterioration and excessive free radical production.

Vegetables and fruits are generally considered low-glycemic carbohydrates because their high roughage content and low caloric levels keep the pancreatic response to a minimum. You should increase your intake of vegetables and (low calorie) fruits, and restrict the grains and refined foods in your diet, if you have any suspicion that you have insulin problems. If you suspect that you have insulin problems, but have not tested positive for them via standard sugar tests, you may still suffer from reactive hypoglycemia. If you are chronically fatigued, this may well be the source of your problems. Cut out all refined foods for three weeks and see if you improve. If so, you can assume you have this condition.

Given all this talk about the "bad" nature of carbohydrates. Don't let yourself forget that you need some carbohydrates for proper brain and colon function, which are best supplied by roughage-rich fruits and vegetables. Minerals from the earth such as calcium and magnesium, and the antioxidant vitamins A, C, E, and selenium also help supply adequate amounts of slow-absorbing glucose for storage in muscles, the liver, and to aid in brain function.

The idea that fish is "brain food" derives not only from its rich DHA and EPA content, but also because fish is an excellent source of protein, which makes glucagon, and is used to mobilize stored glucose. This occurs when the pancreas is activated to secrete glucagon and then mobilizes glycogen stored in the liver and glucose stored in muscle tissues back into the bloodstream. In essence, the pancreas has three jobs: to secrete insulin when it senses carbohydrates coming in, to secrete glucagon when protein enters the body, and to store nutrients, hormones and fats in the cells. When we ingest fish or healthy proteins, our brains work at their most efficient capacity, and receive just the right amount of enzymes when blood glucose is stabilized and insulin is low. Ingesting too many carbohydrates and not enough protein, however, causes insulin to drive glucose levels down, and the body will not be able to make use of any stored glucose. This explains the "brain-dead" feeling that many people experience after large, carbohydrate-rich lunches. Once again, you should not plan to eliminate carbohydrates all together. That response is too far to the left. Rather, choose your carbohydrate sources wisely, and be sure to balance them with adequate levels of protein and fat, in order to keep your glucose levels stable.

If your insulin levels are consistently high, cells will respond by becoming increasingly rigid, a state which hastens cell death. When we are young, cell membranes are fluid and soft, and insulin and other hormones, such as human growth hormone, testosterone, and/or estrogen are easily able to penetrate the cell walls. Nutrients are easy to store within the cells, and therefore they are able to release energy as needed and ensure good tissue health. As we age, however, cell membranes naturally begin to harden (this is a direct result of the affect of insulin on their vital state over time), and communication between hormones and their target cells becomes increasingly difficult. Ironically, as this communication system fails, signals are sent to the hypothalamus indicating a need for even more insulin because glucose is not being stored properly. If the insulin-absorbing system fails entirely, the hypothalamus will call for increased adrenal output, and the adrenal gland, in turn, will secrete the cortisol in an attempt to drive down blood glucose levels. If this is allowed to take place, hypoglycemia or hyperinsulinemia, will result. In extreme cases, adrenal failure may also occur. Do not allow yourself to reach this point! Hypoglycemia is, essentially, the first stage of Type II diabetes. The bottom line is, the more insulin your body must produce the faster you will age.

High glucose levels are deadly. Even though the brain has what is known as the "blood-brain barrier," to keep harmful substances out of the brain, glucose can still enter because of specific glucose receptor-sites. The glucose enters and then causes damage to the ventromedial nucleus (VMN) if levels are too high. These elevated glucose levels eventually lead to permanent nerve and tissue damage.

Protein

Protein is the building block for all bodily tissues and is the foundation of the immune system. Not only is protein a building source, it also has a stabilizing effect on glucose levels. Science has shown us that nitrogen levels, which indicate tissue repair and muscle growth (or the lack thereof) must be maintained at relatively moderate, stable levels throughout the day. If these levels drop sharply, tissue repair is either less effective or muscles begin to atrophy. The best way to maintain these vital levels is to ensure that you are consuming enough protein. As a rule, if you are a very active adult you should take in at least 1 gram of protein per pound of lean body weight every day. This would mean for instance, that a very physically active man weighing 200 pounds, with a body fat percentage of 10%, he would require 180 grams of protein per day. Have your lean muscle mass calculated by a health professional to determine how many grams of protein your body requires. Take your servings of protein, add in calculated amounts of carbohydrates and monounsaturated fats, and divide them into four or five meals per day. Whenever possible, space the meals four hours apart for maximum nutrient absorption and the least amount of insulin response to your caloric intake.

Protein Sources

Before you run out for the health food store to buy buckets of protein powder, or charge to your meat market to buy yourself some fatty steaks, we need to review protein sources for a moment. Pre-modern cultures relied heavily upon wild game, such as buffalo, wild deer and elk for their protein sources. While game meat is naturally lean and free of the hormonal additives present in so many of our modern stock, it is not practical for us to swear off all but game meat in our search for healthy protein sources. Other good sources for protein are lean meats, such as skinless chicken, turkey and the leanest beef, fish (the oilier the better), and eggs (without the yolks). Seek out poultry and beef that were raised organically and "free-range," and not chained to a post or confined in one small area. These animals also should not have been fed steroids, antibiotics, or anything else devised to produce the fattest possible animals in the shortest amount of time. Soy and other vegetable protein sources are acceptable too, but they are much less vital and supply fewer nutrients than meats do. It is my belief that vegetarianism is not the healthiest food choice one can make over the course of a lifetime. It is often difficult for vegetarians and vegans to maintain adequate levels of protein. A lack of protein will lead to caloric deficits, and all too often, increased amounts of carbohydrates or saturated fats end up filling this void. This a double-whammy in terms of fat accumulation and increased insulin levels. We need look no further than our earlier example of the neopaleolithic man to see that eating a diet rich in both meat and vegetables is our best way to maintain muscle mass into our later years, and take maximum advantage of our life span's potential.

As a final thought on protein, I would also caution you against eating fatty meats cooked over an open flame. Many recent studies have shown that open-flame cooking produces potentially carcinogenic enzymes from the meat as the saturated fat drips on the flames and the smoke then sends off a highly carcinogenic group of molecules into the cooking meat.

Fats

Now that we have reviewed proteins and carbohydrates, we must take a look at fats. As previously mentioned, saturated fat, which is derived from animal sources, should be kept to an absolute minimum. Not only does saturated fat increase LDL cholesterol levels, it also contributes to insulin resistance. As a result of our modern domestication techniques of "fattening" our meat supplies, saturated fat levels have climbed far too high in both meat supplies and diary products. Monounsaturated fats, those that are derived from certain nut-plants and other vegetable sources, are much healthier than saturated fats, and should comprise the bulk of your fat intake. Olives and olive oil, some nuts, like almonds; avocados, and canola oil are all good examples of monounsaturated fats. (See "Fats" Graphic G, page 160)

Meal Balancing

Presumably, you have by now calculated your lean body mass and protein requirements. The next step in developing your ideal nutritional plan is to calculate your ideal low-glycemic carbohydrate [14] intake requirements (See Graphic B, page 157). Do this by adding .25X to your lean body mass. To continue with our earlier example of a 200 pound man with 10% body fat (and thus a lean body mass and protein requirement of 180), we would find that his daily carbohydrate requirement would be 225 grams, which should, of course, be eaten in conjunction with proteins and fats, never by themselves, and spread out over four or five small meals.

Finally, you will need to determine your daily monounsaturated fat requirements. Ideally, calories from monounsaturated fats should account for no more than 20% of your total caloric intake for the day. Again, based on these figures we have been using, our subject needs no more than three to four teaspoons of olive oil or canola oil per day. Saturated fats should be avoided whenever possible. In addition to monounsaturated fats, supplementing your diet with molecularly distilled fish oils is also very important. Four to eight grams daily should be sufficient. If you eat in this way, you will ensure that your autocrine (eicosonoid) system's hormonal communications are operating at maximum efficiency, and therefore that your endocrine and paracrine hormones will work to their maximum potential. This, in turn, will increase natural GH receptor sites in the body (slowly reversing cellular aging) and modulating vascular problems, such as high or low blood pressure.

A simple way to remember these portions recommendations while dining out would be to request a lean piece of protein approximately the size and thickness of the palm of your hand. Opening your hand and spreading your fingers out will give you an approximation of the amount of low-glycemic carbohydrates you should consume (mainly green vegetables), and finally, the size of your thumb will provide you a good estimate for calculating your monounsaturated fat allotment for the meal. For dessert, choose a piece of fruit, rather than cake or ice cream.

Do not overeat at any meal, and do not eat fats, carbohydrates, or protein by themselves, as doing so will ultimately compromise the balance of hormone production. By eating frequent, smaller meals, you will keep your nitrogen levels high and therefore secrete more growth hormone, which, as you know, will help you to maintain muscle tissue longer as you age. And finally, by eating in this way, you will be able to keep your body's production of rogue free radicals to a minimum.

Notes:

9

Food & Your Hormones

- **How Food Influences Hormone Production**

Chapter Eighteen:
How Food Influences Hormone Production

As we have discussed, the autocrine system is the underlying hormonal system for all bodily functions because it controls the communication between the body's other two hormonal systems, the endocrine and paracrine. Auto comes from the Greek word avro, meaning self, by oneself, or independently. In endocrinology, autocrine hormones, or "first system" hormones, are often overlooked because of their unique ability to communicate on the cellular level; they do not rely on the bloodstream for communication. Because these messages are conveyed at the untraceable cellular level, they vanish in seconds. The more advanced endocrine and paracrine systems are paid a great deal more attention by doctors and scientists because they leave a trail in the bloodstream. Eicosonoids control all functions on the cellular level, and are the most influenced by which foods you choose. How they are combined, in turn, affects glucagon and insulin production. Glucagon and insulin are autocrine hormones. This is a key point: what we eat affects these hormones tremendously.

To better understand this, we must go back to a time when single-cell organisms existed and communication was only necessary across the cell itself, and simple chemical signals developed to speed this process. As time went by, and organisms started becoming more complex, two or more cells needed to communicate. This very basic intercellular system works relatively well when all of the cells in question are of the same sort, but if there are too many cells in need of the information, the process becomes very slow.

The nervous system developed when the early cell-to-cell communication systems no longer proved adequate for message delivery. The advent of nerves provided a speedy, remote way for organisms to communicate within themselves. Hormones were the next logical step in this communicative process. They enabled cells to develop and react to messages more quickly and accurately than ever before.

Finally, after the development of the nervous system and hormones, the endocrine system emerged. It uses the bloodstream to pass messages, and employs the nervous system as its "feedback loop." Both the paracrine and endocrine hormonal systems are directly influenced in their signals, feedback, and so-called "second messengers," the autocrine hormones eicosonoids. The better one's autocrine hormonal health (cell-to-cell communication) the more freely the other two more complex hormonal systems will work.

Ten Nutritional Rules for Longevity and Building Muscle Mass

1.) Eat four to six small meals per day, in accordance with the ratios given in this book and in The Zone, by Barry Sears. Choose a diet comprised mostly of vegetables and fruits, and rely on them to be your primary sources for carbohydrates. Stay away from a lot of bread and pasta-laden meals. Unlike the plan outlined in The Zone, I do not recommend eating any refined food. Eat raw foods whenever possible.

2.) Eat lean meats, fish, eggs, and whey protein powder for protein sources.

3.) Design a meal program that is comparable to those figures given in the protein section. Your protein intake should be based on one gram per pound of lean mass.

4.) Eat primarily low-glycemic carbohydrates. A glycemic index can be found on the Internet. Find one and stay with that particular one – don't change.

5.) For fats, seek out and use mostly monounsaturated fats, such as some nuts, avocados, olives, olive oil, canola oil, etc. Try to keep saturated fats to a minimum.

6.) Supplement your diet with EPA fish oil capsules.

7.) Don't overeat, even if you missed a meal earlier in the day. Organize each meal this way: protein portions – should be the size and thickness of the palm of your hand. Low-glycemic carbohydrates should take up three times as much space as the protein on your plate. Fats should equal approximately the size of your thumb, or slightly more.

8.) Supplement your diet with the anti-oxidants and minerals listed in the nutritional section of this book and any others that your nutritionist or other health practitioner might recommend. Stay away from so-called "growth supplements."

9.) Drink plenty of water throughout the day.

10.) Stick with it! Discipline is a vital part of your health and fitness plan.

Tests That You Can Do as a Man Over 40 to Identify Possible Food Allergies and/or Low Hormonal Serum Levels

Andropause: What is it? What Do I Do About it?

We all know what menopause is. If your mother (or wife) lived into her late forties and early fifties, I'm sure you saw a difference in her skin-tone; maybe her hair; maybe her personality; maybe all of these and more. Menopause for women is a tough time; it can last for years without much relief. It is a natural biological aging process, however, where the woman slowly looses her ability to ovulate and make eggs – it's evolution's way of giving each women a long enough chance to procreate; then that stage comes to an end. Life is never the same after that.

Although not as potentially devastating and not as overt in symptomology, recently, over the past decade or more, scientists and endocrinologists have been studying and naming a similar stage that men go through. This stage in men has been coined andropause. In short, it means the pausing of making testosterone. This pause is not usually temporary; it's usually permanent, just as with the gradual loss of estrogen and other hormonal balances in women when they go through menopause.

Men often experience sexual impotence, irritability, muscle-mass loss and gradual fatty tissue increase. Much like women's menopause, the male has lost his chance to fertilize a women's egg for reproduction. His life is never the same either.

How Do I Know I Am Experiencing Andropause?

Often times men going through the early stages of andropause will experience some sexual dysfunction; however, as the testosterone levels continue to plummet with age (in most men) the effects can be anything from muscle loss to severe mood swings and loss of natural energy and vitality.

The easiest way to find out the answer to this question is either to ask your family doctor to test your testosterone levels (both "free" and total); or ask him to refer you to an endocrinologists who specializes in hormones and hormonal therapy.

If I Have Below Normal Testosterone, What Can I Do?

Today, thanks to science and research in this area, if you have low testosterone (or hypogonadism – the shrinkage of the testes from a hypo-pituitary axis disruption) you can expect that your doctor will, write a prescription for a testosterone patch, to apply a gel, or take a capsule. Finding the right method is a matter of preference; however, finding the right dosage is altogether a different story.

Not as Easy as it Sounds

Although everyone with chronically low testosterone (or hypogonadism) will eventually reach their biologically correct dosage after months of blood testing and dosage changes; there are a few scientific problems to be aware of.

For one, synthetic testosterone can turn into estrogen – the very opposite of maleness. This occurs when a testosterone gel or patch is applied to the arm or leg area, and since fat cells have a high biological investment in making estrogen from testosterone, often times a dose that seems correct in a one month period; will drop sharply over three months. While applying the gel or patch, the fat cells are helping to convert the testosterone to estrogen – big problem.

The new pills basically do the same thing in another way. As the stomach digests and breaks down the pills, some of the testosterone is lost in this process; while even though the outcome will be an increase in serum testosterone; still, fat cells accumulated on the body will increase the chance of conversion from testosterone to estrogen. I don't advise the use of the pills unless you find that you cannot absorb the testosterone through transdermal gels and/or patches.

This conversion of testosterone to estrogen is not a good thing. The very problems you may have been experiencing in the beginning may become worse if this conversion is prevalent.

The cheapest and most safe way to block this conversion and thus be able to stabilize your testosterone with the aid of your physician is to use a supplement called Chrysin. Chrysin is a natural estrogen blocker and will then allow nearly pure testosterone to be absorbed into the blood stream. Chrysin is not a prescription and can be found at some local health food stores and there are many places on the Internet to buy the product. It shouldn't be more than 20-30 dollars for a months supply; although dosage is purely a trial and error type art – the only science you can be sure of is three consecutive months of elevated testosterone – biologically correct for a person in thier age (and sometimes weight bracket).

Another supplement called D. I. M. (Diinodolymethane) should also be added to your intake to aid in estrogen metabolism.

What About Prostate Cancer and Testosterone Replacement?

Ten years ago, most doctors, especially urologists, would have been against the use of testosterone replacement therapy; however, today, many studies show it may indeed be the loss of testosterone that causes prostate PSA levels to rise and thus be cause for alarm. In a most recent study posted in the New England Journal of Medicine it speaks of this very fact. You are more likely to procreate prostate cancer with low hormonal levels than one's that are biologically correct. When I say biologically correct, I mean standard guidelines that endocrinologist use for people who are in a certain age bracket and have a certain amount of lean muscle mass. Be aware of using too high a dose of testosterone!

Other Factors to Consider

Because the body will often times push the testosterone toward the estrogen side; it is often useful to take DHEA, usually 50 mg. per day as a standard dose. What this does is to merely keep the testosterone building process headed in the right direction – toward Androsteindione and then testosterone. You also will want to make sure you are making enough Estrodiol. This substance is another catalyst in the testosterone production and use cycle. Estrodial can be checked by serum blood or by saliva. It is perhaps DHEA that should be checked by saliva and serum blood. For reasons of accuracy; I would test both ways when it comes to DHEA.

It is important that you are aware of how tricky and permanent testosterone replacement is. Be aware that once you are sure that you have entered into male andropause and you and your doctor decide to begin testosterone replacement therapy; you will be on it synthetically for the rest of your life. It has helped many men in their late forties, fifties, sixties and so on, to regain some muscle mass, energetic vitality and sexual ability.

Tests That You Can Do as a Man Over 40 to Identify Possible Food Allergies and/or Hormonal Low Serum Levels

Andropause

Note: The diagrams below are key elements in the androgenic and steroidogenesis of all vital sexual hormones.

Ideally, the pituitary gland (working in conjunction with the Hypothalmus) should be sending the proper messages to all of the organs involved in the androgenic pathways.

Required Vitamins, Minerals & Supplements

Vitamins

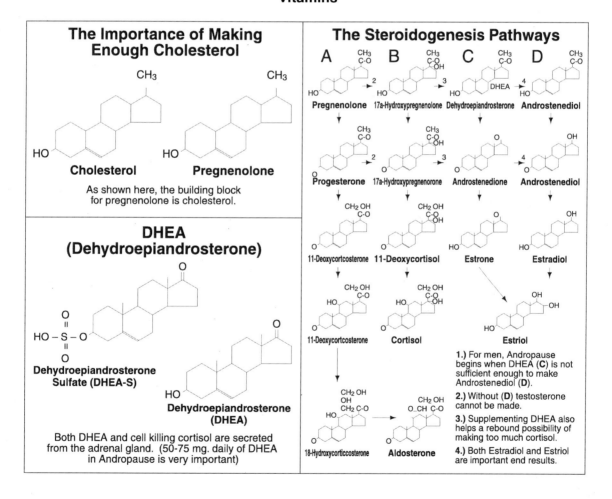

The Importance of Making Enough Cholesterol

Cholesterol   **Pregnenolone**

As shown here, the building block for pregnenolone is cholesterol.

DHEA (Dehydroepiandrosterone)

Dehydroepiandrosterone Sulfate (DHEA-S)

Dehydroepiandrosterone (DHEA)

Both DHEA and cell killing cortisol are secreted from the adrenal gland. (50-75 mg. daily of DHEA in Andropause is very important)

The Steroidogenesis Pathways

A B C D

Pregnenolone   17a-Hydroxypregnenolone   Dehydroepiandrosterone   Androstenediol

Progesterone   17a-Hydroxypregnenorone   Androstenedione   Androstenediol

11-Deoxycortcosterone   11-Deoxycortisol   Estrone   Estradiol

11-Deoxycortcosterone   Cortisol   Estriol

18-Hydroxycorticcosterone   Aldosterone

1.) For men, Andropause begins when DHEA (**C**) is not sufficient enough to make Androstenediol (**D**).

2.) Without (**D**) testosterone cannot be made.

3.) Supplementing DHEA also helps a rebound possibility of making too much cortisol.

4.) Both Estradiol and Estriol are important end results.

A (Beta Carotene), B (Complex), C, D (Unless you live where the sun shines year round), E, Alpha Lipoic Acid

Minerals

Calcium (Coral), Magnesium (Malic Acid), Potassium, Multi-Mineral

Supplements

Co Enzyme Q 10, B-12 (Methylcobalamin), Omega 3 oils (alaskan wild salmon), PH8 (for prostate health), Creatine (powder for weight training only), Pure whey protein, Gookinaid Hydralyte (You can get by going to *www.gookinaid.com*), Somatomed (A Growth Hormone Secretagogue designed to aid in GH output.), Orotine (Orotic Acid - a help in increase of everything from ATP pools to RNA synthesis.)

Vitamins, Minerals & Supplements for Special Circumstances
(This list should be added to the above list for those with Chronic Fatigue, Chronic Fatigue Immune Deficiency Syndrome and/or Fibromyalgia.)

Digestive Enzymes

Betaine, Ultrazyme

Neurosomatic Disorders (CFS/CFIDS)

Magnesium Glycinate Forte, Ultra Lipoic Forte, Homocystrex, Milk Thistle, NAC (N-Acetyl-L-Carnitine, L-Lysine, L-Arginine, 5 HTP (5 Hydroxytryptophan)

For prescription medications, consult your physician. For those with MS, feel free to contact me through my website *www.paulburkefitness.com*. An easy place to find all these supplements is on the web *www.needs.com*

Tests to Ask a Holistic Type, Advanced Thinking Endocrinologist to do:

1.) Free Testosterone --- Blood

2.) Testosterone --- Blood

3.) Growth Hormone --- Blood

4.) DHEA --- Saliva

5.) Estrodiol -- Saliva / Blood

6.) FSH -- Saliva or Blood

7.) LH -- Saliva or Blood

8.) TSH --- Blood

9.) T-4, T-3, T-3R -- Blood

10.) Thyroid Antibodies --- Blood

These are the major test to have done. The main thing you want to remember if any of these levels are low; that you only take what is considered biologically correct for your age. Thyroid results should be taken care of no matter what age you are.

Allergy Tests and Urine Profiles to Check

Many people develop allergies from foods that they have eaten for decades. Food allergies may be subtle, where over years, may cause any problem from IBS to actual degenerative diseases such as MS. Find a clinic that can do both the RAST Test and the Lymphocite Blood tests.

Other Tests to Consider

Urine Analysis Done by Metametrix Labs

This is an entire amino acid, fatty acid and total metabolic organic functional profile. It can be very revealing for ailments that traditional allopathic doctors may not be able to identify with standard blood tests.

Chelation Challenge

This test is done by taking a non-fasting urine sample; then having a 4-5 hour drip of a catalyst used to withdraw metals from your body. Then another urine test immediately after. The comparison of the two reveals that you could have various, possibly toxic levels of metals in tissues or organs.

Author's Note

It is my sincere hope this book has both taught you a great deal and given you a different feeling about your body, how you should feed it, and how best to exercise it. It has been my intent here to bridge the gaps between the old weight training days and today, and between weight training and nutrition; between the best of our Western exercise ideas, with those that have stood the test of time in the East. And, lastly, what we know of our ancestors intelligence to set evolution on a different path.

It is said that experience is life's greatest teacher, I can attest to the validity of that maxim ten times over. But if one does not share one's wisdom and knowledge, what is it worth? This fitness journey of mine has taken me on a real roller-coaster ride of extraordinarily exciting and severely depressing experiences; the most uplifting of these experiences has been the knowledge that I am not alone in this world, that many people will benefit by my life, spent not only working out but also analyzing every different angle, for every different body and body part and metabolism that I have ever been exposed to.

As I am sure you have realized by now, I have no doubts that there are many advantages to weight training and eating in very specific ways, but these ways must not be allowed to consume you. You should be following these ways as a means to express yourself and to stay healthy. Billy Catalina, the owner of the first gym that I ever trained at, used to say, "you should train to live, you shouldn't live to train." Billy was absolutely right. As soon as any of this becomes an obsession, it will turn your life into a one-dimensional state, from which there seems to be no escape.

My best and most honest advice to you is to train hard and give all of this your best effort, and but for a few moments of thought, reflection and notation, and a new consciousness about what you put into your body, leave the rest of it behind when you walk out of the gym's doors. Enjoy whatever else life brings you. Keep your mind open to new ideas and forms. I hope that the knowledge and expertise I have shared with you here has helped to broaden and expand your fitness and nutritional horizons.

It has been an honor and a pleasure to share these thoughts and experiences with you, and I bid you good luck and good health.

Warmest Wishes,

Paul T. Burke

Spencer, Massachusetts
February 24, 2005

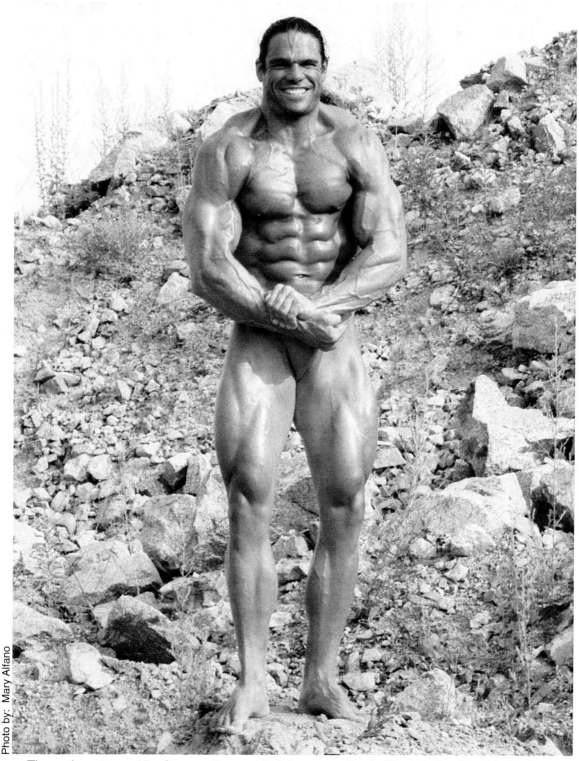

The author at age 40, after creating and training according to "Burke's Law" and just prior to winning a prestigious drug tested contest.

Glossary

Anaerobic Capacity: A level of ultra-strength and endurance forged by using Burke's Law, stimulating muscle to the point of MMS. It is the exercisers' ability to increase both weight and repetitions within any given set, over a course of months, years, decades on any given, or group of exercises.

It was once thought by physiologists that someone is born with so many red fibers and so many white and that this state cannot be changed. However, body builders have proven this theory wrong and Burke's Law uses this as a pillar to create MMS. A person dedicated to Burke's Law, will increase strength and anaerobic capacity as well as changing slow twitch fibers to fast. Of course, only a certain percentage can be converted. However, at the cellular level, a person's mitochondria may allow an increase in the build-up and release of more and more ATP during high intensity weight training. (Mitochondria sustenance and its ability to use ATP as currency is inherited from the mother.)

Biomechanical Leverage Advantage/Disadvantage: A state one finds themselves in when they are using their genetic structural strengths to their advantage. When developing your weight training routine, it is best to find which exercise gives you the greatest biomechanical leverage advantage. If you take ideas from someone who has a specific routine that works well for them, you are probably going to fail because no two structures and physio-kinetic bodies work the same. I have an old rule that dawned on me after years of people asking me how I got my arms so big: "If you have a weak body part and want to find out just one tip that may help you; find someone with the very same problem who has been lifting for years longer than you." They will have a secret for you that may be worth an inch on your biceps. If you have short, flat biceps, never ask a guy who has massive softball biceps because he was given those genes from his parents and chances are they would have been that size and shape no matter what he did. My younger brother has big arms and all he does is carpentry work and sporadic sports. It runs in the family. The idea is to capitalize on the strength of each muscle group as well as finding the way to get to MMS without injury.

Full Range of Motion: An old fallacy that is still believed by trainers and bodybuilders alike that when lifting weights, one has to bring a bar (or dumbbell, or machine handle) "all the way up, and all the way down." I demolish this ideology in the context of "Burke's Law." Everyone should find their "own range of motion" for each exercise.

High Intensity Training: A training method championed by Mike Metzner (former Mr. Universe) who believed that one could create muscle hypertrophy by doing only a few heavy, intense sets for each body part. In my early theories, I began by standing on Metzner's shoulders and was able to quantify and calculate both mathematically and bio-physio-mechanically "Burke's Law." Without meeting and reading Metzner's ideas in the early seventies and early eighties, I would not have been able to write this book at this stage in my career. I would have continued along in this direction, but no paradigm change is done in a vacuum. Throughout history, anyone with an eccentric philosophy is persecuted initially, as was Metzner for he could not articulate what he was experiencing himself. It is only years later when someone else takes the idea and runs with it, as I have here, that the full value can be quantified, made sense in totality and thus used and proven for all to use.

Maximum Muscle Stimulation (MMS): A key ingredient in "Burke's Law". Achieving this state takes continuous moderately heavy repetitions, contracting the muscle intensely, in non-stop fashion until rhythmic, fluid, stable repetitions can no longer be generated by the focus muscle group. The faster you can achieve MMS, the more progress you will make in your effort to achieve muscle hypertrophy.

Muscle Elongation: A state that a weight trained muscle is in when in perfect fitness health. To reach this, a weight trained muscle (which when hypertrophied will cause shortening) must be relaxed and stretched. It is a physiological kinetic fallacy (and fantasy) that a muscle can be stretched when lifting weights and stretching on a mat and forcing your muscles to "stretch" is least effective and worse yet, possibly injurious to men over 40 years old. The best forms of passive stretching are swimming, Yoga, and Tai Chi. Walking is also a valuable stretching exercise provided your form is correct.

Muscle Hypertrophy: The end result of stimulating the muscle (usually with weights, or anaerobic type exercises) creating tiny micro-tares, which grow back slightly larger assuming that proper rest, nutrients and hormones have been supplied for cellular growth. Of course Muscle Atrophy is the exact opposite: This is when there is a reduction in both size and strength. Muscle Atrophy is a Biological Marker of Aging and therefore weight training done properly should be done lifelong.

Myofascia: Myofascia is a thin sheath that covers all the muscles and tendons of the body. The white, thin layers on chicken breast between the skin and the white meat is myofascia. In experiments scientist have shown that the stress hormone cortisol can increase myofascia thickness, which can lead to many maladies including Myofascia Pain Syndrome and Fibromyalgia.

Neutral Hand Position: When the wrist turns upward and clockwise, but only until it is in alignment with the forearms. In this position your thumbs will be facing up. One usually does V-bar low pulley rows with a "neutral" position.

The Old Paradigm: The term I use to describe the training ideology of the past 50 years. It is not that I throw this entire ideology out, I merely scientifically challenge and change this ideology. Burke's Law is a "Neo-Paradigm."

Pronation: When the wrist or ankle is directed downward. A pronated wrist will leave your hand in a position to do wide-gripped Pull-ups; or reverse-grip "Zotman" curls.

Supination: The ability of a joint to turn upward and clockwise. Both the wrist and ankle can supinate. During concentration curls for the arm biceps, supination of the wrist (and hand) is essential so as to work toward a "peaked" biceps. (There is never a reason to supinate your ankle; if fact, if anything you want to build the calves only in tight up-and-down motions so as to prevent supination of the ankle, which, under weight will cause a severe sprain.)

Bibliography

Anatomical Chart Company. 1998. "The World's Best Anatomical Charts," Skokie, IL.

Austad, S.N. 1997. Why We Age. New York: John Wiley & Sons.

Baynes, J. W., and V.M. Monnier, Eds. 1989. The Maillard Reaction in Aging, Diabetes, and Nutrition. Alan R. Liss, New York:

Bernardis, L.L., and P.J. Davis. 1996. "Aging and the Hypothalamus." Physical Behavior (59: 523-536).

Burke, Paul T. "Food and Hormonal Communication." Exercise for Men Only.

_____. "The Markers of Aging." Exercise For Men Only.

_____. "Muscular Arms for the Man Over 40." Exercise For Men Only.

_____. "Nutritional News: Understanding Creatine." Men's Exercise.

_____. "The Paradox of Exercise." Exercise For Men Only.

_____. "Slowing Down The Aging Process." Exercise for Men Only.

_____. "The Synergy of Food and Exercise." Exercise For Men Only.

_____. "Understanding the Biological Markers of Aging." Exercise For Men Only.

_____. "Understanding energy In Relationship to Exercise." Exercise For Men Only.

_____. "Youthful Energy." Exercise For Men Only.

_____. "The Zone Diet, Part I." Men's Exercise.

_____. "The Zone Diet, Part II." Men's Exercise.

Butler, George, Haines. 1975. Pumping Iron, New York: Simon & Schuster.

Butler, George, and Gerome Gary. 2003. Pumping Iron, The 25th Anniversary

Edition. New York: Simon & Schuster.

Butler, Tom, and George Gaines. 1974. Pumping Iron. New York: Simon & Schuster.

Columbo, Franco and George Fels. 1978. Coming on Strong, Chicago: Contemporary Books.

_____. 1979. Winning, Body Building, Chicago: Contemporary Books.

Columbo, Franco, D.C., with Richard Tyler, 1979. Chicago: Contemporary Books.

Crist, D. M., G.T. Peake, P.A. Eagan, and D.L. Waters. 1988. "Body composition response to exogenenous GH during training in highly conditioned adults." Journal of Applied Physiology 65: 579-584.

Erasmus, Udo. 1993. Fats That Heal, Fats That Kill: The Complete Guide to Fats, Oils, Cholesterol and Human Health. Burnaby, BC, Canada: Alive Books.

Felig, P., J.D. Baxter, and L.A. Frohman. 1995. Endocrinology and Aging, 3rd. Ed. New York: McGraw-Hill.

Leigh, Wendy. 1990. Arnold: An Unauthorized Biography. Congdon & Weed, Inc.

Little, William, H.W. Fowler, and Jessie Coulins. 1973. The Oxford English Dictionary. London: Oxford UP.

Murray, Michael T., N.D., 1991. Encyclopedia of Natural Medicine. Rocklin, CA: Prima Publishing.

_____. 1996. Encyclopedia of Nutritional Supplements. Rocklin, CA: Prima Publishing.

Parr, T. 1996. "Insulin exposure controls the rate of mammalian aging." Mechanics of Aging and Development (88: 75-82).

Roth, J.S., M. Gluck, R.S. Yalow, and S.A. Berson. 1964. "The influence of blood glucose on the plasma concentration of growth hormone." Diabetes (13: 335-361).

Schonfield, J.G. 1970. "Prostaglandin E1 and the release of growth hormone in vitro." Nature (228: 179).

Schwarzenegger, Arnold. 1977. Arnold: The Education of A Body Builder. New York: Simon & Schuster.

_____ and Bill Dobbins. 1985. The Encyclopedia of Modern Bodybuilding, New York: Simon & Schuster.

Sears, Barry. 1999, The Anti-Aging Zone, New York: Harper Collins.

_____. 1996. The Zone. New York: Harper Collins.

"Superoxide Dimutase (SOD)" Medline Plus, National Library of Medicine Web site, http://www.nlm.nih.gov/medlineplus/mplusdictionary.html

Thissen, J.P., J.M. Ketelslegers, and L.E. Underwood. 1994. "Nutrition regulation of the insulin-like growth factors." Endocrine Review (15: 80-101).

Willoughby, David P. and George R. 1947. The Complete Guide to Muscular

Measurements. Montreal, Quebec: Weider Pub.

Teihard de Chardin, The Phenomenon of Man, translated by Bernard Wall, forwarded by Julian Huxley, William Collins & Sons Ltd., London 1959.

W.S. Penn, editor, The Telling of the World, Native American Stories and Art, Stewart, Tabori & Chang, New York, 1993

Albert Einstein, Relativity, Crown Publishers Inc., 1961.

Teihard de Chardin, The Phenomenon of Man, translated by Bernard Wall, forwarded by Julian Huxley, William Collins & Sons Ltd., London 1959.

W.S. Penn, editor, The Telling of the World, Native American Stories and Art, Stewart, Tabori & Chang, New York, 1993

Steve Jones, Robert Martin, David Pilbeam. Executive Editor, Sarah Bunney, Forward by Richard Dawkins. The Cambridge Encyclopedia of Human Evolution, Cambridge University Press, 1992.

R.D. Martin, Primates Origin and Evolution, Princeton University Press, 1990.

J. Reader, Missing Links: The Hunt for Earliest Man, Penguin Books, London, 1998.
R. Milner, The Encyclopedia of Evolution, Humanity's Search for its Origins, New York,

1990.

R.E. Passingham, The Human Primate, Oxford and San Fransico, 1982.

I. Tattersall, Encyclopedia of Human Evolution and Prehistory, Garland Press, New York and London, 1988.

M.W. Stricken, Evolution, Jones and Bartlette, Boston, 1990.

J. Gowlette, Ascent to Civilization: The Archeology of Early Humans, Maidenhead and New York: McGraw Hill, 1993.

J. Diamond, The Third Chimpanzee, Harper Collins, New York, 1998

Jared Diamond, Guns, Germs, and Steel, W.W. Norton & Co., New York 1992.

Kent Flannery, "The origins of agriculture," Annual Reviews of Anthropology 2:271-310.

Jack Harlan, Crops and Man, 2nd. ed. (Madison, Wis. American Society of Agronomy, 1992.

Sun Bear, Waban Wind, Dreaming with the Wheel, Simon & Schuster, New York, 1994

Thomas E. Mails, The Mystic Warriors Of The Plains, Mallard Press, 1972.

Natalie Curtis, The Indians Book, Authentic Native American Legends, Lore&Music, Bonanza Books, 1987.

Duane Champagne, Chronology Of Native North American History, Gale Research Inc., 1994.

Timothy Severen, Vanishing Primitive Man, American Heritage Publishing, New York, 1973

W.S. Penn, The Telling of The World, A Fair Street/Welcome Book, New York, 1990.

Felig, P., J.D. Baxter and L.A. Frohman. Endocrinology and Aging, 3rd. ed. McGraw-Hill, New York, NY (1995).

Austad, S.N. Why We Age. John Wiley & Sons, New York, NY (1997).

Baynes, J. W., and V.M. Monnier, eds. The Maillard Reaction in Aging, Diabetes, and

Nutrition. Alan R. Liss, New York (1989).

Sears, B. The Anti-Aging Zone, Harper Collins, New York, NY (1999).

Bernardis, L.L., and P.J. Davis. "Aging and the Hypothalamus." Physical Behavior 59: 523-536 (1996).

Parr, T. "Insulin exposure controls the rate of mammalian aging." Mechanics of Aging and Development 88: 75-82 (1996).

Crist, D. M., G.T. Peake, P.A. Eagan, and D.L. Waters. "Body composition response to exogenenous GH during training in highly conditioned adults." Journal of Applied Physiology 65: 579-584 (1988).

Roth, J.S., M. Gluck, R.S. Yalow, and S.A. Berson. "The influence of blood glucose on the plasma concentration of growth hormone." Diabetes 13: 335-361 (1964).

Schonfield, J.G. "Prostaglandin E1 and the release of growth hormone in vitro." Nature 228: 179 (1970).

Thissen, J.P., J.M. Ketelslegers, and L.E. Underwood. "Nutrition regulation of the insulin-like growth factors." Endocrine Review 15: 80-101

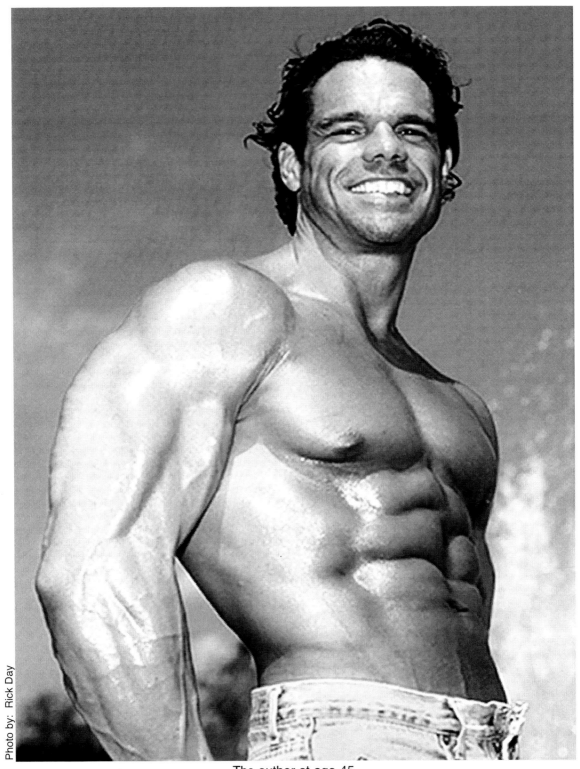

The author at age 45.
Photo: Courtesy of Chelo Publishing

Appendix A
My Workout Routine and Dietary Habits

I have chosen to include my own workout routine and dietary habits here only as a rough guide for you to use. You must remember, however, that each person needs to develop his own routines and diet, based on what is best for him. Also, bear in mind that I have been training with weights for almost 40 years, and have spent a lifetime exploring and modifying the theory of Maximum Muscle Stimulation. My routine should not be your routine, Do not feel that your routine should mimic mine. To give you a bit of context, I am six feet tall and weigh 210 pounds. I have approximately 6-8% body fat, and eat roughly 190 grams of lean protein per day. Based on the ratios outlined earlier in the book, you can estimate my daily carbohydrates intake, which fats I eat, and how I supplement my diet.

For the sake of easy understanding, I will organize my routine based on a sample two-week period.

Monday: I awake feeling well rested and full of glucose and stored glycogen (in the liver). I have not worked out with weights in three days, and the only exercise I have done was to walk a mile two days ago. Before working out I take some creatine mixed with cold water or green tea. I also drink cold water or cold green tea during my workouts.

I begin my routine with a combination of cables and dumbbells. I use three thick Lifeline cables to do low rows for the inside of my back. This has done a great deal to help me achieve a good balance in my back thickness and its width. Using these cables has also allowed me to bring my shoulders back to a proper anatomical position. (Too many years of heavy bench pressing had caused my shoulders to slope, the overuse was too much for my body, and everything was pulled forward as a result). I do 20 perfect, heavy squeezing repetitions with the cables, and then lie on the floor to do as many cable curls with both arms as possible. If I were at a gym, I would opt to perform as many preacher curls as I could, until achieving total muscle failure. I have found that cables can be the perfect replacement for weights, and they have allowed me to drastically reduce my instance of injury. Muscles only grow under the weight of heavy contractions, so cables are just as effective as weights although for contraction, the resistance of weights does promote more and faster muscle hypertrophy, if used accordingly. The so called "negative rep" is virtually useless. Control the weight, but work on the "positive contractions".

After finishing with the cables, I move immediately on to as many heavy flat bench dumbbell presses as I can without stopping. I have not rested to this point. I do 15 non-stop reps with the heavy dumbbells and then rest, sip some water, and repeat the group of sets again. I will do this for four rounds, until my back, chest, and arms are pumped to their maximum. Though I am exhausted at this point. I have just completed in 15 minutes the same amount of sets, reps and weight that would take most people at least an hour. Please note – you should not try this until you have built your anaerobic capacity a great deal. For this rapid training to be effective, you need to have converted a lot of fibers from fast to slow twitch, a process that takes years. Think of my example here as something towards which you should be working. Even now, however, you can train in a heavy, hard, fast, intense way to the point of exhaustion without injury.

I would now rest for a minute, have some more water, and try to catch my breath. Once I am rested, I will do a set of triceps pushdowns to failure, without stopping, using a set of cable crossovers for my pecs. Then I will finish with some concentration curls, again, each done until failure. Like with the earlier exercises, I will go from set to set without stopping until I have finished four complete cycles. I have now exhausted every muscle in my upper body in 20 minutes. My muscles have now been pumped to the point where my biceps are 20" in circumference, my forearms are 16", my abdominals can easily be seen, my chest is engorged with blood, and my waist is about 31-32". There is no need for me to work out any more. With so much of my blood circulating through my upper body, it is not uncommon for me to need to sit down because my legs feel weak. Again, only use my routine here as an example of what to work toward – if you try this too soon, you will either lose your breath and turn the lifting into an aerobic exercise of futility, or you will not be able to lift enough to reach MMS; or, you could end up with some severe medical emergency. I recommend that you work two muscle groups on any given day.

Tuesday: I will do nothing physical today. I am sore, and I know I need to rest more than anything.

Wednesday: Today I will swim for 40 minutes. Twenty minutes will be spent swimming free-style, and the other 20 minutes I will spend doing the breast stroke as quickly as I can. Immediately after leaving the pool I will feel heavy, but know I will feel energized later in the day.

Thursday: If it is a nice day, I will walk a mile or a mile and a half, first walking uphill as hard as I can, and then back down more slowly, yet still briskly.

Friday: I take the day off from training.

Saturday: I begin the day with my creatine supplement, and then work my legs. This is hard for me, but I know that everyone has areas that are harder for them to work than others. I warm up with a few hundred pounds on a leg press machine.

Depending on how I feel, I will add anywhere from 500-800 pounds, and then rest until my heart rate is down to 90 beats per minute. Once recovered, I begin the reps, pushing almost to the top, and then I go back down as fast as I can, until I am buried and must push with all my might to get the platform up and locked. My thighs begin to swell at this point, and, depending on how much they swell, I may or may not do another set. More than likely, if I have done somewhere in the vicinity 800-1,000 pounds 25-30 times without stopping, I will not do another set. Remember I am moving these reps faster than most people can count, and as my ATP levels begin to wane, only my mind can force the last five presses. Usually, there is no need to do anymore, for my legs will be exhausted.

As a finishing exercise, I will do two sets each of leg extensions and sets of leg curls in "super set" fashion. Then, I use the weight that was on the leg press to work my calves until I can no longer move them. I will know when I am done because it will be very difficult for me to walk. My entire lower body routine will have taken approximately 15 minutes.

Sunday: I rest.

Monday: I will go swimming again, using the same routine as the previous week.

Tuesday: I will walk for a mile to mile and a half.

Wednesday: I will either rest or work my upper body, depending on how I feel.

Thursday: I will work my upper body, if I did not work it on Wednesday.

It sounds so simple, and that is the way it should be, but to get to this level, it takes dedication, belief, and years of hard work.

My eating habits follow the guidelines I set forth in the book. My breakfast is usually five egg whites, one egg yolk, and a piece of fruit. I take all of my vitamins in the morning, and drink a protein drink of pure whey protein and water.

Two hours after breakfast, I will have some turkey and a salad.

Three hours after the second meal, I will have a piece of grilled salmon, lots of steamed broccoli, some asparagus and some pecans. I often use hummus as a dressing for my vegetables. I will finish the meal off with a small piece of fruit.

Three hours later, I have a protein drink and a piece of fruit, maybe some nuts.

Dinner is the same as lunch (salmon and vegetables, often times fresh corn on the cob or rice, rarely).

For nighttime snacking, I usually choose one or two Zone bars, or some yogurt with grapes and nuts.

Every day I drink at least a gallon of fluid. I usually drink water or green tea and throughout the day I drink a rehydration drink called Gookinaid which has a perfect ratio of potassium/sodium calcium/magnesium and is also low in sugar. I try to eat sushi once or twice a week and often juice vegetables, drinking 4 to 6 oz. every other day. I use raw, unpasteurized butter and use a tiny amount of canola oil to cook with.

I eat and drink this way all of the time. If I go out to eat, I order a filet with broccoli and a salad, or plain grilled salmon, broccoli and a bowl of fruit for dessert. Remember the simple rule of thumb: a lean piece of protein should be the size and thickness of the palm of your hand, green vegetable servings should equal the size of your entire hand (with fingers) spread out, and a piece of fruit is your best choice for dessert. You can use a teaspoon of olive oil or canola oil, or a pat of butter once in a while. It's quite simple when you think about it and, like anything; it is dedication that will give you the results you desire.

During other periods I may break my body parts as such:

Workout Day One	**Chest:**	Six sets, three sets of two different exercises.
	Triceps:	Six sets, three sets of two different exercises.
Workout Day Four	**Back:**	Eight sets, four sets of two different exercises.
	Biceps:	Six sets, two sets of three different exercises
Workout Day Six	**Legs:**	Three sets of multi-muscle group exercises. Two sets of leg curls. Two sets of leg extensions. One set working calves to failure.

Appendix B
Sample Assessment of a Recent Client

The following is a reprint of an assessment I recently conducted for one of my clients. Reading through it might be helpful to you, as you seek to formulate your own diet and fitness regimen.

Dear Bill,

Welcome to the "Paul Burke Over 40 Fitness" family! I have read over your recently completed nutrition and fitness questionnaire, and was quite interested in your responses. I have never before come across anyone who practices kumdo. I congratulate you on your choice of a martial art for exercise, as I believe that they offer the sort of valuable mind/body/spirit connection that many of our Western gyms and health clubs often overlook. As you may know, I am a great believer in combining the best of Eastern and Western fitness modalities.

Along with an ideal fitness regimen, I will strive to help you develop the best possible diet, so that you can shed body fat and gain muscle mass and muscle tone. To do this, as you may have guessed, you will have to change some of your ways. Most people are not "balanced" in their fitness or dietary habits; to this end, I will give you a routine to follow, one designed with your best health and interest in mind, and together we can bring you into balance. In developing your routine, I will do my best to address your ailments, injuries, and diet allergies, and will then create with you an entire lifestyle change – one that is not too dramatic, but is different enough to help you achieve your goals.

To begin, it is obvious to me that you are currently pursuing a very asymmetrical fitness regime. Without a doubt, the number one way to maintain your fitness and physiological/biomechanical integrity is to cross-train. Cross-training is something that you probably did as child, if you played football, baseball, basketball, volleyball, etc, either in an official or unofficial capacity. As we age, we tend to "find what we are good at," and stick with it, and asymmetrical fitness programs are the natural result of such behavior. Kumdo sounds like a tough, contact sport/art form, and while I am not encouraging you to give it up by any means, its very nature seems to demand that you pair it with cross-training. Once you begin a cross-training program, you can expect to get rid of some of your injuries, and also loose body fat, gain muscle size and tone, and eliminate the fear of an early death.

Your pulse and blood pressure are all relatively good. Your systolic level is a bit high, but that will come down in time. It's odd that your diastolic level is 70, but I assume that is from the drugs you are taking. You will have to explain more to me about those drugs. Sleep apnea is related to your weight, I am sure of that. I am unfamiliar with what GERD is, so you will need to tell me more about it and how it works for you.

Thinking, now, of the injuries you mentioned in your questionnaire, most specifically your fractured calcuanus bone, it is imperative that you begin working both sides of your lower legs equally at the gym. Your resulting weight loss will also help your injury, as you build muscle and achieve an overall slimming effect. Your injury won't magically go away, but it will feel much better. The bursitis that you speak of is both mechanical and dietary in nature, and I will address it in this exercise plan, as well as in your diet. Your arthritis in L-4-5 can be attributed to the weight you are carrying, all without the requisite lumbar strength to support it. This will be addressed in your fitness routine. Your knee problem will probably go away in a month or so, once I explain to you how to rehabilitate it in the gym.

I encourage you to read the articles I have published in the "Fitness Lifestyles" section of my Web site, and also in the various magazines I write for (a guide to these can also be found on my Web site). I also recommend that you read articles and books such as The Anti-Aging Zone, by Barry Sears; Eat 4 Your Blood Type, by Dr. Peter D'Adamo; and The Third Chimpanzee, by Jared Diamond. If you would like additional reading recommendations, please don't hesitate to contact me. The goal here is to expose you to several dietary philosophies, so that you can see how I came to build my own. You cannot know too much about your own body, and by exposing yourself to as many different perspectives as possible, you will find yourself in a more powerful position than the cry for help that I heard when reading through your questionnaire.

Turning briefly, now, to your dietary issues, as noted on your questionnaire, I must say, it is not wise for you to consume saturated fat, such as the cheese that you report you eat, in spite of the knowledge that you are more than likely lactose intolerant. Saturated fat, which is found in all animal meats, increases insulin resistance, which in turn, is part of the problem with your glucose regulation. You might be interested in reading "Fats that Heal, Fats That Kill," by Udo Urasmus. It will give you a good sense of the crucial role played by fats in our overall health status.

Your questionnaire answers tell me that you are currently carrying too much fat around your waist. At 6', with an 8" wrist, your waist should not exceed 36." This measurement is a goal for you to shoot for. As you lose excess fat, you will also experience an increased capacity for glucose regulation and lipid ratio corrections. When you are carrying extra fat, you are at a greater risk for developing Type II diabetes and arterial sclerosis. Your new diet will help correct this problem. Be prepared – you will need to cut out saturated fats (like cheese) and refined foods, such as bread, pasta, fried foods, etc. Instead, choose to eat fresh salmon and skinless chicken; this will help you immensely.

The above issues are the elements of your questionnaire that really stuck out as I read over it. Rest assured, I have devised for you a nutrition program that will incorporate your current good habits (such as kumdo) with new ones to address your ailments, weight, and lifestyle. I have also constructed a fitness plan for you, which we will implement and modify, as needed, over time.

Your New Diet

I have identified 10 simple rules for your new diet. If you follow them, you will be well on your way to better health.

1.) Begin eating smaller meals, but eat at least four times per day.

2.) Download a glycemic Index chart from the Internet for future reference.

3.) Study the glycemic index and identify all of the vegetables (and fruits) you like that have a rating of 60 or below. (No more fried foods!)

4.) Eat 8 ounces of lean protein at each meal (a list of acceptable protein sources can be found below - page 200 of this book). For you, I recommend fish, skinless chicken, tuna, and turkey breasts, rarely lean beef. You have to cut out the cheese.

5.) Always determine how many grams of protein are in your meal's selection. (You can either download a list of protein gram/caloric ratios, or buy a booklet with this information. I will provide approximate portion size information here, but to be exact, and be part of the process, you still need to spend the time to do it yourself. By doing this work yourself, you will be able to internalize the process more fully.

6.) Always determine how many low-glycemic carbohydrates you need to eat each time you consume protein. (To do this, take your grams of protein and multiply it by .25.) Mix up your vegetable intake – don't eat the same ones all the time. Implementation of this rule may be hard for you at first, you might experience lethargy, headaches, variation in bowel movements, etc., but these difficulties will correct themselves in 7-10 days.

7.) You may add one tablespoon of canola or olive oil, avocado, or plain nuts (not roasted) to each meal. This fat source should not exceed 150 calories.

8.) A basic rule of thumb, especially if eating out, is to ask for a serving of plain grilled fish or chicken the size and thickness of the palm of your hand. Eat plain, steamed low glycemic carbohydrates in a serving about the size of your entire hand spread out, or the size of a medium size plate. (You may find that you will need two plates at some meals, one for protein and another for vegetables.) Then, have a small amount of fat from the list at the end of this section.

9.) For dessert, you may have an apple or pear, some grapes, or other low-glycemic carbohydrates, but nothing else for now!

10.) Again, eat four meals per day, one every four to five hours.

When you begin following this diet, you will notice a marked increase in your insulin level stability and health; this is because you will be eating in a manner pleasing to the pancreas. The pancreas' job is to regulate blood glucose and to secrete glucagon.

Glucagon is a hormone that is secreted as a response to ingesting protein. Simply put, it mobilizes blood sugar. Low-glycemic carbohydrates act as a counterbalance to glucagon, and help maintain blood sugar equilibrium, therefore whenever you are taking in protein, you will also need to consume the appropriate amount of low-glycemic carbohydrates. Keep in mind the formula for calculating these ratios and you will be fine.

You may be wondering why I recommend only the low-glycemic carbohydrates. It is simple – any carbohydrates that have

Best Proteins	Best Vegetables	Best Fats	Best Fruits
Salmon	All Greens	Raw Almonds	Apples
Skinless Chicken	Peppers	Raw Hazelnuts	Pears
Hard Boiled Egg Whites	Asparagus	Raw Macadamia Nuts	Strawberries
Skinless Turkey	Tomatos	Avocados	Blueberries
Whitefish	All Squash	Olive Oil	Blackberries
Soy Beans	Yams	Canola Oil	Honeydew
Low-Fat Beef	Sweet Potatoes	Pine Nuts	Cantaloupe
Ham	Any Other Vegetable Below 60 on The Glycemic Index	Olives	Cantaloupe
Tuna		Pecans	Cantaloupe
Yogurt (Plain, if Lactose Intolerant)			Cantaloupe

been processed (high-glycemic carbs) cause the pancreas to secrete too much insulin. The glycemic Index predicts how much and how fast the pancreas will or should secrete insulin. Insulin is paradoxical in that we need it to penetrate cells to facilitate the storage of hormones and micro-and-macronutrients, but, if our bodies overproduce it, hypoglycemia will result. An excess of insulin will drive blood glucose levels down too low, and then, over time, the brain's hypothalamus will instruct the adrenal glands to secrete cortisol to lower insulin levels. From here, a vicious cycle emerges, and you will find yourself with too little insulin, too much cortisol, and your cells will not be permeable enough to allow for the much-needed hormonal and nutrient penetration. We need insulin to live, but if we make too much or not enough, we will die. Luckily, by pursuing a low-glycemic carbohydrate-rich diet that is also high in lean protein, this "worst case scenario" is avoidable and even reversible. You may not have any of these problems now, but believe me, they are on the horizon, unless you change your eating habits.

The foods listed in the chart are the safest for you to build your initial diet around. Use hummus or tiny amounts of olive oil/vinaigrette to dress your vegetables. Do not use any oils except those listed above. In addition to addressing insulin levels, this diet will also help alleviate the bursitis you report.

Keep The Following Things in Mind:

Grill or poach all of your proteins, and steam all of your vegetables.

Strive to be accurate with your 8-ounce servings of protein, remember to balance them with the appropriate amounts of low-glycemic carbohydrates, and use only a small amount of the aforementioned oils or fats.

Eat only the fruits listed, and only two desserts in a day.

Refined foods are like a drug; the more you eat them, the more of them your body will crave. After you have been on this diet for a while, the cravings you experience for fried foods or breads will subside.

To help reduce cravings, try brushing your teeth after each meal. The taste of the toothpaste will help make your cravings go away.

As a final dietary note, I recommend that you have a food lymphocyte allergy test performed, to see if you have resistance to any foods other than dairy.

Your New Workout

Before beginning this, or any other, new workout, you should schedule a check-up with a cardiologist, and be sure to let the doctor know you are beginning a new exercise program which will include weight training, aerobic activity such as walking and swimming, and that you will continue with your kumdo practice, and may also be adding yoga to your routine.

Until your weight has begun to drop, I would hold off on other, more intense exercises like basketball. Do not add more intense activity to your routine until your resting pulse rate and blood pressure levels are more consistent than they are at present.

Begin your routine with three weekly 30-minute walking sessions. I also recommend that you join a gym, so that you can add some very basic weight lifting exercises to your work out plan. Only use the weight machines, stay away from free weights for now – this will help you avoid overdoing it.

What follows is a good guide for how a typical training week should flow.

Monday: Do one or two light sets of each of the following exercises on a machine. Only complete 10 reps with a light weight that you can handle easily. The main goal on this first day is simply to get the feel of the machines and exercises. Concentrate today on the chest press, incline chest press, seated fly machine, and vertical chest press.

Ask one of the trainers at the gym to demonstrate the machines for you, and then make certain that you are using them properly. Keep your feet flat on the floor, and concentrate on maintaining parallel and perpendicular lines when using the machines. When you extend your arms, they should form a straight line across your upper chest, for example. Hand spacing is usually a shoulder's width apart, and foot spacing is usually hip width. Your knees should always move above the feet in unison. If you do not maintain this form, you risk injuring yourself.

Tuesday: Take the day off. Do not exercise at all.

Wednesday: Walk for 30 minutes.

Thursday: Return to the gym, and do one or two 10 rep sets on one of the following machines: lat pull-downs; seated pulls, rear deltoids, lats; low pulley row; or a pull-up machine (or do standard pull-ups if you can do them without help. If you need help, use a Gravitron or similar machine to help counterbalance your body weight. When performing pull-ups of any kind, hold the bar two fist lengths beyond your shoulders.

Concentrate on your form, nothing else. Use a light weight for all of these exercises, don't struggle. You are in the form building stage now. Keep that in mind – I cannot stress enough that proper form requires that you keep all joints, and limbs at right angles or parallel, relative to the machines.

Friday: Take the day off from exercising, but do research as to where you can go swimming or take yoga classes. Do one of these the following day,

Saturday: Either swim or do yoga. You cannot substitute kumdo for this, as we are trying here to form new fitness habits. Your body is already primed for kumdo, and we are trying, with this new workout plan, to help you achieve a more balanced fitness regimen.

Sunday: Walk for 30 minutes.

Monday: Return to the gym and work on one or two easy sets of the following: hack squats, horizontal leg squats (which are good for knee rehabilitation, if they feel "good"). Incline leg presses, leg extensions (which, together with incline leg presses are ideal for knee rehabilitation), standing leg curls, and lying leg curls. To help work the back of your calves, do some calf raises, both standing and seated. For the front of the calves, practice some frontal toe raises, which will help your soleus (the broad, flat muscle that helps to flex the ankle and depress the sole of the foot). If you have found a place to swim, do so today.

Swimming is an important companion exercise to weight training. By lifting, you are making your muscles stronger, which is a good thing, but they also will become shorter. Soon your muscles will begin to hypertrophy (grow), and you will need to work to lengthen them as much as possible. Swimming is the best way to achieve this; alternate freestyle with the breaststroke. Swimming allows your body to relax while in motion, and the stretching motions of the strokes will lengthen the muscles while you are building cardiovascular stamina. I hope you will give this a try. You should swim as often as you lift weights, and for the same length of time. If you can't swim, yoga is the next best thing. Yoga will help you balance the kumdo portions of your workout plan. For now, limit your kumdo to one or two days out of ten. The days to practice your kumdo would be those when you are not lifting weights or taking a day off (a day for walking would be ideal).

This new exercise plan is a lot for you to deal with, and I don't want to overwhelm you, so I will stop here. But, I want a full report of your diet and fitness activities in two weeks, and we will work form there. This will be a long, hard, but fun adventure Steven; please don't expect instant results. The need for a perfect form is of the greatest essence when performing these new exercises. Listen, watch, and learn. Get your muscles to get into a "groove" when performing your sets.   This applies to swimming strokes (have a pro watch you) and yoga as well.

Don't think in terms of "workouts per week" as most people do, just follow the plan I have outlined, and be certain to rest whenever you feel sore. Do not train with weights if you are sore anywhere. At first, this may be often, but your body will soon become used to it.

Finally, on another day, I want you to have a trainer to teach you how to do the following:

Seated Triceps machine

Triceps Pushdowns

Triceps with a rope or a dumbbell, overhead

Standing barbell curl

Scott, or Preacher Curls

One arm concentration curls.

Walk the day after you learn to do these, and keep up the swimming and yoga practice!

When you have done everything listed above for two weeks, e-mail me and tell me what you have done, in detail. Don't forget; keep track of which exercises you are doing and which ones felt good and not so good. Note which ones help or hurt, or anything else noticeable. I want to know everything that goes on, so that I will know how best to help you from that point. Your report will give me a good idea of your physiological fitness. Follow these plans as if your life depends upon it – because it does. I will help you in any way that I can, but you have to do the work. Remember, this is a new journey; it won't be easy, but the rewards are great.

Appendix C
Sample Questions and Answers
From My Column in "Exercise For Men Only"

The following questions and answers are a sampling of those that I have received from readers of my "Exercise For Men Only" column. I have chosen them for inclusion here because they address many of the concerns shared by so many people in this age group.

Paul,
I have had two total shoulder replacements thus my ability to perform heavy lifting chest exercises is limited. I cannot perform any heavy overhead motions to increase my shoulder size. I have competed in the INBF twice recently, and both times placed 5th, due to my asymmetrical back, shoulders, and arms. What exercises can you recommend for me? PS, Steve Downs (the "EMO" editor) suggested several rotator cuff strengthening exercises that have helped to stabilize my shoulders and allow me to lift heavier weights with my chest muscles.

Carl

Carl,
I admire you for having the courage to compete after receiving shoulder replacements – this is great! I suggest you look at your problem in a new light. Given your shoulder limitations, I do not recommend that you attempt extremely heavy shoulder exercises, however, if the replacements were fitted properly, they should not limit your range of motion. Therefore, there is no reason that you cannot develop your chest, deltoids, back, and arms to balance out your physique. Make this problem the driving force that turns you into next year's champion. How? It's a matter of imagination and focus. Find a comfortable weight and focus on your form, perfect it, and then concentrate on the muscles you are working like never before. Get inside those muscles every rep. Imagine them growing, like small foothills turning into mountains. Try doing 20-30 reps in a set instead of the standard 6-12. You might even seek to develop your own exercise that no one else has ever thought of. Look outside the "normal" range of perception about exercise. You are limited only to the extent that you think you are limited. If you focus enough within your new seemingly-confined parameters, you will see the world of muscle development open up to you. These constraining factors will then become your great assets because you will be concentrating harder and raising your level of consciousness for the task at hand. This is your opportunity to find the rainbow at the edge of this thunderstorm. It is your opportunity to build a better physique for yourself than you would have if these obstacles had never presented themselves.

Paul,

I am soon to be 46 and for about 10 months now I have been training for an hour three times per week. I divide these sessions in half, with 30 minutes each spent on cardio and weight training. I belong to a gym, so I have access to most equipment. Unfortunately, the staff at my gym is not very knowledgeable. What would you suggest to guide my training? I am approximately 20 pounds overweight (5'9", 200 lbs) and would like to build upper body mass.

Ed

Ed,

I think you are right on track with the amount of time you are spending in the gym. How efficient you are with that time is key. I recommend that you spend your time perfecting your form for each exercise to the very best of your ability. In weight training, I have come to learn, perfect form added to the ability to pump the muscle continuously until failure, is far more important than the amount of weight being used, a the number of reps performed, or the amount of time spent in the gym. One set completed with perfect form, comprised by ten or twelve smooth, non-stop reps is worth two weeks of struggling against heavy weights, squirming, and yelling for attention. Focus on Form, concentration, and your intensity. Find someone in your gym who makes weight training look like riding a bike and mimic them; or watch the movie "Pumping Iron" and watch Arnold perform his concentration curls and low-pulley rows. Notice that he doesn't cheat, he keeps the weight moving until the end, and he makes it look easy. You want to be able to look in the mirror and watch yourself pump reps just like that. Perfect a smooth, fluid, rhythmic type of rep, with a moderate weight that allows you to push (or pull) for ten, then squeeze out one or two more without stopping, and you will be done. Concentrate on your muscle the entire time. Developing a perfect form will build muscle memory and allow you to concentrate on the continuous pumping of the muscle. If there is a "key" to training, this is it. Perform three or four sets per muscle group, not counting warm ups, and stick to your diet, and you will make progress; it is that simple.

Paul,

One of your areas of expertise is anti-aging technology, please explain to me what this is and how it can help my workouts. I currently train six times per week in an effort to hold back the hands of time. One area that I need to focus on is abdominals. Any insight would be appreciated.

Rick

Rick,

We use the phrase "anti-aging technology" to highlight the fact that certain biological mechanisms of aging can be effectively identified and slowed down by some dietary and exercise modifications. If you are exercising with weights six times per week, you are, in my opinion, overdoing it. In fact, by exercising at this level of intensity, you run the very real risk of regressing or staying the same in terms of muscle-building, and you also may be causing more cellular damage than if you didn't exercise at all. According to a Harvard study, there is a point where exercise brings not only diminishing returns, but also outright negative effects.

If you are training naturally, meaning without the aid of steroids or growth hormone, there is no reason to work out six times a week with weights. Rather, I advise you to work out three times per week with weights (working each body part just once, skipping a day in between), and do 40 minutes of brisk walking or light aerobic exercise the other three days. This is not only a very effective strategy for developing muscle, it will also help you to lower your body fat and ensure overall balanced health.

If you are concerned about developing your abs, it will interest you to know that the most important component of so-called "ab development" is one's diet. The fewer refined foods (pastas, breads, sugars, juice drinks, dried fruits, etc.), and saturated fats that you consume, the more body fat you will burn, and the more you will be able to see your abdominal muscles. Monounsaturated fats such as olives, some nuts, and avocados, are fine in moderation. In many cases, a person's abs are already "developed" but are hidden under a layer of fat. To help reduce any layers of fat you may have in this area, I recommend doing a couple of sets of leg raises and crunches twice a week at the end of your workout. Remember, however, it is your diet that will contribute more to your abdominal "development" than any long and torturous ab routine.

Paul,

I am 61 years old and have been bodybuilding for at least 10 years with no results that I can brag about. Recently, I mentioned this to my doctor, he ran a blood test, and determined that I have very low testosterone. He gave me a shot but nothing has happened! Do you have any recommendations for what I might do to bring about some improvement in my appearance? Could my very low testosterone level be responsible for my poor showing regarding bodybuilding? Are higher levels necessary for high achievement?

Tom

Tom,

Your question is one of great complexity; however, I will try to answer it as best I can. It would be helpful to know what "low" testosterone is in your case. Is it presently less than 200? The range for "normal" is 300-1200. Ideally, it would be wonderful to know what your levels were the ages of 20, 30, 40, 45, and 50; however, this is unrealistic in your case. It is quite possible that your particular range was "low" even when you were young. In other words, a low "normal" level (300-400) may have been your testosterone "high." If this were the case, knowing this would be very instructive if your levels are presently 250-300, for example, as that "low" reading wouldn't be so low for you.

I am assuming that your doctor gave you an injection of oil-based testosterone. There are three things to keep in mind concerning these sorts of shots. First, it usually takes 3-6 injections of 100 mg (per cc) before protein anabolism begins. Meaning, muscle hypertrophy and the other anabolic effects (such as increased libido) won't occur for about a month, if you are receiving weekly injections. Second, I don't think elevating your testosterone should be your first course of action. When you inject testosterone, your pituitary gland is likely to go into a relatively dormant state. Once the hypothalamus senses higher levels of (synthetic) testosterone in the blood, the pituitary will not send any more signals to the testes to produce testosterone (See Graphic E, page 155). In other words, your own testosterone levels will slowly diminish. Unless you want to take an injection every week for the rest of your life, I would not choose this method as a first treatment to enhance testosterone. Rather, I see it as a last resort. Third, it is very common for men your age to have lower levels of testosterone, and for good reason. Elevated testosterone levels often have a negative effect on the prostate gland. If you have even a hint of prostate problems (such as an elevated PSA level) you are playing with fire by injecting testosterone. (Some new studies show contradictory evidence.)

There are a few ways to elevate testosterone levels naturally. Two simple ways are to exercise with weights and to eat more protein. I assume you are doing both of these. There are also a few natural products on the market that enhance testosterone production. If you go to a good health supplement store, you will be able to purchase any number of products that have this effect. Try a few of these products and see what you think. These supplements enhance testosterone production, while injections of testosterone, though highly effective at first, will eventually bring your natural testosterone production to a halt. Finally, you can still stimulate muscle growth even with low testosterone levels.

I advise you to work out with weights only three times per week, focusing on each muscle or muscle grouping just once. Stick to 8-12 reps in the upper body, and 12-20 in the lower. Work toward nice, rhythmic sets that bring the muscle to fatigue without causing you to shake or move your body around while performing the sets. Also, stick to multi-joint exercises like the bench, leg, and shoulder presses, pull-ups, barbell curls, etc. Avoid so-called "isolated" movements.

I also recommend eating one gram of protein per pound of lean body mass. Have a body fat percentage test done at your gym or doctor's office to determine how much lean mass you carry. I would divide this protein requirement into four or five small meals of protein, carbohydrates, and fats, and strive to include a lot of fresh fruits and vegetables in your diet. Stay away from anything refined, such as bread, pasta, sugar, or fruit juice, and seek out monounsaturated fats from nuts, olives, and avocados. Cut out animal fats as much as possible.

Testosterone is only one component of muscle building. I suggest you read as many studies and books on the subject as you can before you continue. There is no a simple solution, and mishandling the situation could ultimately cause many problems.

Footnote References

[1] Lead shot was added and removed by taking off a small cap on each end of the barbell. It was difficult to be certain how accurate the balance was – making his lifting even more amazing.

[2] Cyr lived 1863-1912. Sandow lived 1868-1925.

[3] Over the head lifting was made an Olympic event because the IOC deemed it more "athletic" and crowd-pleasing than other forms of weightlifting.

[4] We'll get into this much more as we move along through history of the sport, and then move into the specifics of Burke's Law.

[5] See http://www.bodybuilding.com/fun/galanis9.htm for more in-depth information on ATP and how it is used.

[6] For more information, see http://www.feldenkrais.com/

[7] The AC joint is formed where the acromion (top of the wing bone, or scapula) connects to the collar bone, or clavicle

[8] Chronically high levels of insulin bring on endocrine stress.

[9] The autocrine system regulates cell migration.

[10] SOD is "metal-containing antioxidant enzyme that reduces potentially harmful free radicals of oxygen formed during normal metabolic cell processes to oxygen and hydrogen peroxide."   For more information, see the Medline Plus home page at the National Library of Medicine, http://www.nlm.nih.gov/medlineplus/mplusdictionary.html

[11] Glucagon is, primarily a glucose mobilizer.

[12] You can find the glycemic index on the Internet, or in nutritional books at your local bookstore.
[13] Those with this natural pancreatic "buffer" tend to be descended from the earliest groups of pre-agrarian humans.   Those of northern European ancestry, Native

Americans, most African-Americans, however, usually have not been blessed with this natural buffer.

[14] For future reference, those carbohydrates under 60 on the glycemic index are primarily fruits and vegetables.

Index

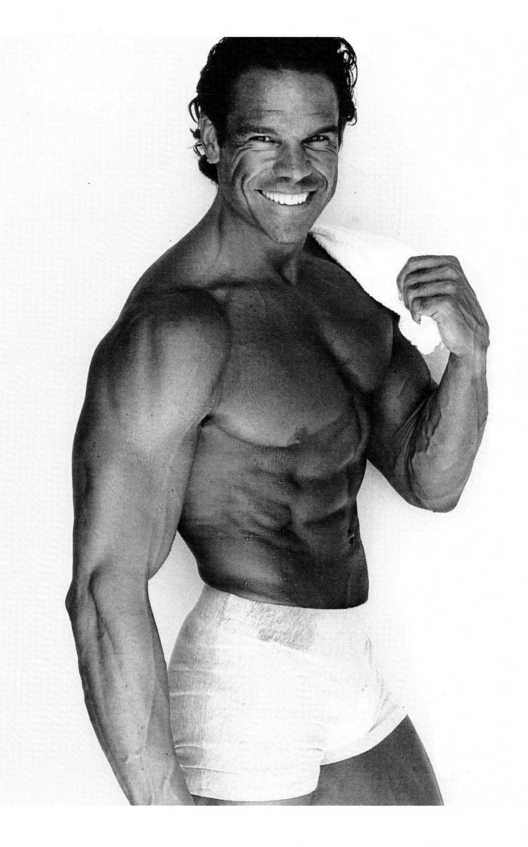

About The Author

Paul Burke has a Master's degree in Integrated Studies from Cambridge College, in Cambridge, MA. He is a former bodybuilding champion, arm wrestling champion, an actor, member of the Screen Actors Guild, and a professor. He owns a successful business, and was decorated by the United States Air Force (USAF) for Meritorious Service, and won the Sikorsky Helicopter Rescue Award for his role in a life saving mission. While in the Air Force, he devised and implemented the first weight-training program for use by the USAF (Europe). The most defining element of his life, he says, has been the job he held with a traveling circus and carnival after he ran away from home at the age of 16. Without that background, he reports, he never could have written this book.

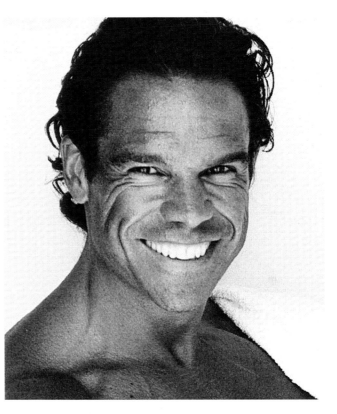

Mr. Burke operates the Web site Paul Burke's Over 40 Fitness & Nutrition, which can be found at http://www.paulburkefitness.com.